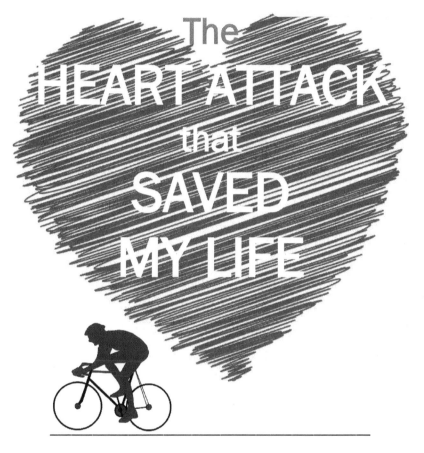

The HEART ATTACK that SAVED MY LIFE

AND MY RIDE BACK TO HEALTH

RUSSELL C. ANDERSON
with VALERIE N. ANDERSON

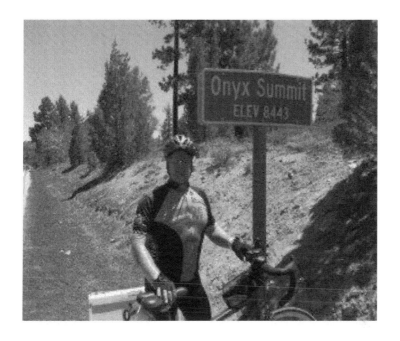

Russ at the highest elevation through the mountains above our
city during a Ride Around the Bear event.

iv

Dedication

The song, "Living On A Prayer" by Bon Jovi has been our song since Valerie and I became engaged in 1987, and it is still an important part of our marriage! Our entire adventure continues to be "Living On A Prayer." I want to acknowledge the many who have helped along the way, including: Dr. Steven Wilson, Ride Yourself Fit, Yucaipa Bike Center, Redlands Cyclery, Don's Bikes, Mike Quinlin, and Mark. I also dedicate this book to my son, James, who encouraged me and became a cyclist with me, which brought joy to my heart. Finally, and most importantly, I dedicate this book to my wife, Valerie, who continues to support my cycling and is still my best friend! I love her, very much and look forward to the journey that is ahead of us!

Chapter 1

Life Before

January 28, 2001: the day my life changed forever. That was the day that at 39 years old, I had a heart attack. Of course, it didn't start on that day; it actually began a long time before that, growing up in the Midwest.

I had a very good childhood, with a brother and wonderful parents in Illinois. My dad had a great job and provided well for his family; my mom was a stay-at-home mom, who was a very good cook. She had dinner on the table every night between 5:00 and 6:00 p.m. My mom prepared wonderful meals, full of flavor, from different ethnic backgrounds, but leaned towards Italian meals. Many of the foods she prepared were extremely delicious; however, they had high fat content, cholesterol and calories. She always made a point to include a vegetable with each dinner, but I was very good at avoiding them. Despite being a heavy child, my

1

parents emphasized eating everything on my plate.

I was always a pudgy kid, short and stocky, as I like to call it. My Mother was an excellent cook, but she cooked foods that were heavy and full of fat, and my parents told me to eat all of the food on my plate, because there were starving kids in China that did not have food to eat. As my wife pointed out after we got married, and I told our son that, she asked me if any of the food my Mother cooked made its way to China. I thought about it and realized that it was just a ruse to get me to eat everything on my plate. In school, I was always the last to be picked for teams, and I later wondered why my parents would have a fat boy eat everything on his plate!

My parents got my brother and I involved in the YMCA's Indian Guides, going off-roading, camping and playing some sports, but I was always a pudgy kid. My parents tried to help me lose weight, but it was never really on my mind. My priorities were pretty much fun, motorcycles, school, and in that order. This went on for most of my childhood and into my teen years, until I met a friend in high school, who told me about weight lifting.

So, I did just that – I started weight lifting. I gained 20 pounds in less than a month in muscle and re-shaped my body, but my eating habits were still very poor.

In the coming years, I relocated to Southern California, finished high school, and made new friends, but continued in my playful, poor-eating habit lifestyle. I wasn't really active in any sports, other than occasionally playing Frisbee or softball. After

2

years of this, I married a wonderful woman, Valerie, who already had a great son named James, and we started a life together. Valerie and I bought a mobile home in lovely Yucaipa, a small city pressed up against the tall mountains that separated the Los Angeles sprawl from the far-emptier desert. Yucaipa sits high enough in the foothills (at about 2,500 ft. elevation) to give us distinct seasons and cleaner air than most of SoCal.

Because my wife and I are Christians who also enjoy motorcycles, we became involved in the Christian Motorcyclists Association (CMA). We joined a band that played at the motorcycle rallies, churches and events, and traveled with this band for almost three years. The CMA is a tremendous organization that preaches the Gospel to people who ride motorcycles from all different walks of life. A great bunch of people; however, they really did like to eat. In fact, they had a saying, "'Til We Eat Again!" This did not help my health, because I was not making good choices on what to eat, and I ate all the time. Still, no serious exercise, except to my forearm, raising my fork up and down to my mouth.

During the time we were in the band, our son was involved in soccer, which also took up a lot of our time. We signed him up with the city's soccer league, and we were committed to taking him to two practices a week and going to his games every Saturday.

In 1989, I started working at Cal-Mesa Steel, a local steel distributor and fabricator. The band we were in dissolved and we continued to be very involved in our son's soccer.

We had attended four different churches that helped us to grow in our Christian walk during the first 12 years of our marriage. Up to this point, I really believed I had the typical diet of the American man – a lot of fast food and little exercise. In late 2000, I noticed the first symptoms that something was wrong.

Chapter 2

Uh oh.

What was that?

While I was at work one day in November of 2000, I noticed a streak going across my left eyeball. I had never seen anything like this before. I called my wife and told her I needed to go see an eye doctor. We made an appointment, and my eyes checked out fine, but my blood pressure was very high. I then went and saw my family doctor, Dr. Steven (Steve) Wilson. He saw my high blood pressure and did an EKG. What it showed was that my heart was enlarged, due to the high blood pressure. An enlarged heart is different from a large heart. In an enlarged heart, the ventricles reduce in size, due to the thick walls of the enlarged heart, making the heart less efficient. Athletes, such as runners, cyclists and swimmers, may have a large heart with large ventricles that works efficiently, due to their cardiovascular training.

Dr. Wilson put me on blood pressure medicine, which lowered my blood pressure and reduced the enlargement of the heart, but some unseen damage was done. About a month and a half later, I was helping at a clean-up day at our church. There was an extra piece of property next to the church that needed to be cleaned of debris and collected items over the years. It was very dirty and dusty. One of the items that needed to be moved was an old, broken down drinking fountain. Two men were looking at it, trying to figure out how to move it, because it was very heavy. Being very strong, but not very wise, I picked it up by myself and carried it to a recycling bin. It felt like it was 175 pounds. When I set it down and stood up, I felt a pain going up each side of my neck, which I had never felt before. I thought it was simply a respiratory problem, due to being around a lot of dust, so I continued to work. I did not feel any chest pain.

I continued to help, and the next thing we moved were cement parking blocks. As I continued to work and picked up a cement parking block, I felt the pain again, along each side of my throat. At this point I felt that something was wrong, but I still suspected it was merely due to breathing dust or maybe that I had an allergy to something. At that point, I left and went home.

In the coming days at work, since I worked at a steel company and lifting heavy steel is required, I began feeling jaw pain, again.

I still did not have any chest pain. The severity of the pain increased each time it occurred. During that week, I went to see my doctor, and he discovered my blood pressure was extremely high. I did not tell my doctor about the severe pain I was having in my neck and jaw. I know I was afraid to find out that it might be something more serious.

That Saturday, I had more pain in my jaw, but I did not tell my wife, because I did not want her to worry. However, Sunday morning, January 28, 2001, I woke up with sever pain in my throat and jaw. It felt as though my jaw was being crushed, and I still did not have any chest pain.

My wife called a friend of ours, who is a cardiac Nurse, and she recommended we go to the emergency room. I foolishly thought that taking a shower would help me feel better and relieve some of the pain. While I was taking a shower, my wife got ready, so she could take me to the hospital. As soon as I got out of the shower, my wife hurried me to get dressed and rushed me to the emergency room. NOTE: One of our mistakes was not calling for an ambulance, which should be done any time a person thinks they are having a life-threatening issue. I should have called an ambulance, since I was informed by our friend that it may be my heart.

Once I was at the emergency room, my wife got me checked in and I had to wait for about 15 minutes before I was seen by a nurse. I was initially being seen by a nurse, who took my vital signs and checked my oxygen levels. My blood pressure was 220/150 and they took me right away to a bed. I was then hooked up to get an EKG. The doctor was given the EKG Report at the nurse's station outside of my area. My wife went to the doctor and asked him how it looked, and he told her, "Your husband is having a heart attack right now!"

The doctor then came into the room and told me that I was having a heart attack right then, and the nurses came from every direction and began hooking me up to IVs and spraying nitroglycerine into my mouth. The nitroglycerine did not immediately work, but as soon as the Heparin drip began, the pain began to subside. At this point, I wasn't scared, because I was still in denial. I could not believe that I was having a heart attack and told the nurse, "I can't be having a heart attack, I'm 39." She told me that they see people a lot younger in the emergency room having heart attacks.

My wife stepped out of the emergency room momentarily to call our son and our pastor to inform them of my situation. She was shaking and was a little bewildered when she was calling our son, because she was watching it all transpire right in front of her and she told me it was happening in slow motion. Valerie told me later that she finally knew what surreal meant! She told me that as soon as the doctor left the nurse's station, nurses, techs, and an x-ray technician all came from different directions and converged around my bed. I had a chest x-ray, I was hooked up to an IV and two nurses were trying to give me nitroglycerin. I kept trying to sit up, so the nitro kept missing getting into my mouth. My wife was standing at the foot of the hospital bed, and when I would not listen to the nurses, she told me, "If you don't lay down and do what you're supposed to…," so I laid down. I knew she meant business!

While I was still in the emergency room, they did a blood test, which showed cardiac enzymes, which is an indicator of a heart attack, and they scheduled me for an angiogram. I was then taken to ICU, so they could continue to monitor my health and heart.

The next day, I was taken down to have an angiogram. This procedure is where they run a camera up through an artery by the groin, because it is a very large artery that can handle this procedure. The camera is run up to the heart to see if there are any blockages. One blockage was found, but it was only blocked 45 percent. I was told that this could be treated with medication and change of diet. They had a policy of not putting stents in arteries unless there was a 50% or greater blockage. I was in the hospital for five days and was sent home that Friday feeling fine and was now about to be off of work for two months to recuperate, which was not making me happy. I enjoy working and hated the thought of sitting at home, but the two months began.

Russell C. Anderson and Valerie N. Anderson

Chapter 3

Now What?

The first thing we had to do after I came home was go grocery shopping. This was quite an excursion, because we read every label of every item we picked up in the grocery store to check for fat, saturated fat and salt content. It took us two and a half hours to finish our grocery shopping. Despite being at a grocery store known for their healthier items, it was still necessary to read every label, because even though a product is labeled "vegetarian" it can still have an extreme amount of salt or fat.

When Valerie and I got home from the store, we went through the cupboards and the refrigerator and had to throw out anything that would be harmful after my heart attack. We knew that we were throwing away money but it was important for us to have me feed on the best diet/eating plan I could, so I would avoid another heart attack. It was also very frustrating to think that I would not be able

11

to eat some of the same things that I was used to eating, but the sacrifice was worth it, because I did not want to have to go through any of this again!

My mind was now thinking about what was ahead for the next two months. I was told to rest. I've been a hyperactive person since the day I was born. I was so active, that my parents had to take me to the emergency room multiple times for carelessness. Now, I was facing two months of rest and relaxation that I did not know how to accomplish. The thought of resting and not being able to be as active as I had been was bothering me tremendously. I was wondering if I would be able to enjoy my life ever again.

It seemed overwhelming to me, the change that would have to take place in my life. Together, Valerie and I purged the house of high fat foods, high sugar foods, high sodium foods and greasy foods. Not only did my eating habits need to drastically change, but I also needed to change the way I thought, because I was always worrying and stressing, which contributed to my high blood pressure. This was especially difficult, since worrying and stressing had been a habit of mine since I was very young. I did not know how to shut off the thoughts that caused my anxiety. I always envied those people who were very calm in stressful situations. I have never been the 007 type – calm under any circumstance!

I also needed to start exercising, and we all know about the dreaded "E" word. It was hard to know where to begin. It was amazing to me how working and the daily routines replaced any thought of exercise. Looking ahead to the next two months seemed daunting, but I knew I had to stay busy because I was determined to go back to work.

During those two months, I did stay busy helping with housework – vacuuming, dishes, laundry, cooking – boy did Valerie love that!!! However, despite staying busy in the house, and resting, I was still not exercising the way I was told to by my doctors. So, I made a decision to begin walking.

The first time I went for a walk, I went up the street from our house and made it to the first light pole, about 200 feet, but just doing that was scary, because I was afraid that if I went farther, something would happen and would not get back home. So, I turned around, and went back home to try another day, because I was short of breath. Every time I felt short of breath or pain of any kind, I was afraid that something was happening again. My doctor reassured me that the twinges of pain and slight stabbing pains were nerve-ending pains and they normally occurred after this type of procedure, and the worrying about it could do more harm than what I was feeling. He encouraged me to stay active.

The next day, I went for my second walk and was determined to go to the second light pole, which was about 300 feet from the house. Our street has a slight incline, so it is a little bit harder to walk up the street. I did make it to the second light pole! I felt a sense of accomplishment. Over the next couple of days, I only walked to the second light pole, only a little faster. By the following week, I was walking to the third and fourth light poles, and eventually, around our block. My energy was increasing, and I was feeling hopeful!

Up at the top of our street there is a small canyon, like a wash. I started walking down into that – it is quite hilly and steep. This was a bit scary to me, but I was getting bored just walking on the street. I started covering more and more ground during my walks, and I was seeing animals and scenery that I had not noticed before. I was actually having quite a bit of fun.

Finally, in late March, I was cleared to go back to work. Right now, I have to say, one of the worst parts of this entire experience was having two months off of work! I like my job and I enjoy working. It felt great to get back to work! Although I had to take it easy and could not lift over 10 pounds, which is difficult at a steel yard, I managed to do my job. Everybody at my work was very supportive and encouraging. They were all curious about how I was feeling and wanted to do whatever they could to help.

Everything was going just fine, working, walking, eating right, resting, until the day before my 40th birthday, which was April 16th. I felt something familiar – I felt throat and chest pain. Very reluctantly, I told my boss about how I was feeling and he sent me to the emergency room. I called Valerie and told her I was heading to the emergency room, but not to come, because she was at a new job and I would probably be okay. Actually, I was scared to death!

I was put on a gurney and a nurse was taking my blood

pressure, which was very high, again. While I was lying there feeling very scared, I saw Valerie walk in. Please excuse the pun – my heart leaped! I was so glad to see my best friend. It is amazing that no matter what you're going through, when you have a buddy with you, a best friend, it all seems much better and not so scary.

While there, the cardiologist decided that since all of the equipment was ready, I would be given a stress test. I was hooked to an EKG and had to walk on a treadmill for six minutes with increasing elevation. When my heart rate was significantly higher, the doctor took me off of the treadmill and examined me with an ultrasound machine to see how my heart was reacting to the stress. Valerie and I got to see the valve working in my heart and it was amazing to see how my heart was beating. The doctor informed me that my heart was okay. He felt the pain was probably from something else – like a pulled muscle. This was good news, because I had told Valerie that I was not going to spend my birthday, which was the next day, in the hospital!

I went home and celebrated my 40th birthday with my wife and son with joy that my heart was doing well. Valerie gave me a carrying case for my telescope accessories, which was a great gift. I have an interest in astronomy, as well. I like to look at God's fingerprints!

I continued with my daily routine, working, walking, resting, and eating right for about three more weeks. Then I had a bad day.

Russell C. Anderson and Valerie N. Anderson

Chapter 4

I Can't Believe This is Happening to Me

I woke up on May 9, 2001 and this time, I knew something was wrong. I was feeling chest pain and jaw pain and I was terrified. I knew this time it would be more than just simply laying in the hospital bed with an IV in my arm. I called my boss and told him what I was feeling, what was going on and that I was going to the emergency room. He was concerned and asked me to let him know what was going on.

Valerie and I went to the emergency room. Upon arriving at the emergency room, I was examined, did an EKG, blood enzyme test and x-rays and scheduled an angiogram, just like the first one. At this point, I was extremely fearful – I knew this was not a respiratory problem. I knew something was going to happen, I just didn't know what to expect. The angiogram showed a 95% blockage of the artery that had been shown as 45% blocked back in January. I was admitted to the hospital and taken up to ICU.

In ICU it was decided that, since Redlands Community Hospital did not have a cardiac unit, I would be taken to Loma Linda University Medical Center (LLUMC), which is about 15 miles west of where we lived, to have a stent put into my artery. I was thinking about injuries I had over the years, punching my hand through a glass door, and the glass piercing through my hand and severing some nerves and seeing the blood squirting out of my hand like a squirt gun. Or, the time I was on a friend's dirt bike, road too close to a trailer and caught the corner of the fender with my right foot and tore my foot open and seeing the blood oozing out of my shoe. This seemed more terrifying than those accidents, because I could feel pain from deep inside, but I could not see what was going on. They were taking me to LLUMC, one of the best hospitals in the world to fix what was wrong inside of me. The fact that I needed to go to that stature of hospital scared me. Valerie was in the room with me the next morning when the EMT's arrived to transport me. They took me by ambulance and Valerie drove to meet the ambulance at the hospital. She stayed calm through this whole event, but I knew she was scared inside. She didn't want me to see any fear, because she didn't want me to worry. She kept telling me that God was going to take care of me, that He would guide the doctors during the procedure and I was going to be okay.

I was taken up to my room to await being taken on the gurney down to the operating room. When I was wheeled down for the procedure, I was put onto the table, where I came to the realization that I was completely naked. I was feeling very self-conscious, but then I realized, "This ain't anything they haven't seen before." So I basically told myself, "Oh, well." In time, there was a staff of doctors and nurses around me, and they said they were going to give me an angioplasty. The doctor explained to me that an angioplasty was basically an angiogram, but it had a balloon on the end with a stainless-steel mesh that the doctor explained looked like the spring that comes in a ballpoint pen. He said it was about three quarters of an inch and made of titanium.

He told me I could watch the entire procedure on a monitor right above by head. I said, "You mean I'm going to be awake?" He said that they prefer that, so I could tell them what I was feeling. However, they did give me a pill to relax me – praise God!

They entered into an artery by my groin and maneuvered the mechanism up through my body to the clogged artery in my heart. I saw the wire with a balloon on the end, the angioplasty tool, very clearly on the screen above my head, going through my artery to the narrowed point of the artery. Fortunately, they had given me some medication so I would relax, but I was still awake, so I wasn't feeling great fear; I was amazed that I could watch this in live time.

The doctor pointed out exactly what was happening as the wire moved through my body. When it reached the artery, the doctor told me that he was going to give me a heart attack by inflating the balloon. I literally saw the balloon inflate; I felt an extreme pain in my chest and passed out.

During this entire procedure Valerie was in the waiting room, praying and trying to stay calm, knowing that I was in good hands. When the procedure was over, they informed her it had gone well and they were taking me up to my room. She was elated and knew that God had helped me come out of it okay.

Almost exactly 24 hours after the stent was put in, I woke up. A nurse came in and gave me a piece of paper that explained what I could and could not eat. She stressed that I eat vegetables, fruits, walnuts and lean meats. By now, it was common sense for me to stay away from greasy, fried, fatty foods. Exercise was also emphasized. I was told by a nurse that there are three heart-healthy exercises, running, swimming and cycling. All of them are highly cardiovascular, but a truth is that they each have a problem. Running pounds joints and can cause damage. Swimming needs a pool and not everyone has a pool in their backyard or can afford a membership where there is a pool and in cycling, you can crash – and I have crashed. After I was given this information, along with dietary recommendations, I was released on Friday, May 11, 2001.

I was ordered to stay home and rest for two weeks, which was a lot better than two months. However, I could not believe that this had happened to me. There I was, 40 years old, a man that at one time was able to bench 300 pounds, almost always active and was now relying on prescriptions and procedures to keep me alive. "How the hell did I get here?"

Russell C. Anderson and Valerie N. Anderson

Chapter 5

Depression and Resolve

I was sent home the day after I had a stent put in my artery to open it up and keep the blood flowing properly through my heart. I felt very depressed, because I could not believe I had another "heart event" and had to get a stent put in my heart. It was difficult to grasp the real severity of the situation.

I had to stay home for two weeks this time, so I began walking again, but not as diligently, and I took care of things around the house, because Valerie was working and was tired when she got home each night. I felt hopeless! I really felt that my life would now be going from procedure to procedure and medication to medication from then on, and I didn't like that the staff at our local pharmacy knew me! I really didn't want to be well known at the pharmacy! I really questioned whether I would be healthy and active ever again; "Will I ever feel normal again?"

At my lowest point, when I was sitting in our garage, I was looking out across the driveway and saw my son, James, walking toward me. He asked, "Whatcha doing, Dad?" My feelings just came out, and I said, "I'm just taking up space and killing time." I don't think my words registered with James as to how badly I was feeling. I felt that my life would not amount to anything; I would be restricted in everything I would do from that point on. I would not be able to lift more than 10 pounds, not be able to enjoy any food that I normally enjoyed, such as steak and potatoes; I wouldn't be able to travel for fear of having another heart attack; it all seemed pointless and a waste of life.

It really was a hopeless statement that I said to my son, but when I told my wife what I said to James, she completely understood what I meant and was encouraging me with all of the possibilities with my heart being healthier than it was before the heart attack. After talking with Valerie, I felt a little better. I was trying to grasp the positive aspects that were ahead of me, as opposed to the discouraging side of resting for two weeks, on top of the two months I had to rest after the initial heart attack. Why did they call this second one a "heart episode?" It wasn't an "episode." I was a bonified heart attack that required a stent; an invasion into my body to put something in an artery that looked like a spring out of a pen. Why do they wait until arteries are 50 percent clogged before doing anything; why didn't they help my arteries when they were 45 percent clogged? Why wait? Why give the body the chance to clog the artery even more, so a person can have pain, discomfort, sadness, frustration, disappointment, hopelessness and depression? What was the point of waiting? Why didn't God heal my arteries from the heart attack in January, so I wouldn't have to go through what I went through? What was wrong with me that the one artery clogged five percent more to cause me more grief? I didn't have any answers to any of my questions!

I went ahead and called my pastor, Don Hinkle, who had had a heart attack and bypass surgery, because I felt he would understand what I was feeling and might be able to help me understand my feelings and get a better outlook on my life.

My pastor came by the next day to visit me. We sat in the same spot in the garage where I had been sitting several days before. I was anxious and nervous about sharing my feelings with my pastor. Where I was a man who shared my feelings with my wife because we are best friends and talk about anything and everything, sharing my feelings with another man was very different. I had seen myself as a strong man, emotionally and physically, but since the heart attack I felt weak mentally and physically. All kinds of thoughts ran through my head – could I still provide for my wife and son? What kind of future would I have with them? Could I still do my job and give it my all? Would I let the company down that had been so good to me for so long? Would I lose my job? Would we have to sell the house and move into something smaller and more affordable? Would I lose my life insurance because I had a heart attack? Would my health insurance have me pay higher co-payments for every doctor visit? On and on and on the thoughts would go through my head and haunt me. I really did not know how to express everything; I thought I would sound like a raving lunatic. Would I have a great future with my wife, doing the things we were dreaming of and talking about or just a mediocre future? Was I going to let her down? She would tell me how much she loved how strong I was; would she see me as less of a man now? I wondered if I might have to go on disability and live a life less than productive and less than I wanted to live. Would I be able to be a true leader and mentor of my family? Would I be able to be a contribution to society? Would I be able to teach my son how to be a strong man of true integrity and strength in everything that could come his way? Would my wife look at me differently? Would Valerie see me as weak when I used to be very strong? Would she want to stay by my side, even if I couldn't do the things that I used to be able to accomplish for our future? Would Valerie feel safe around me and feel I could protect her as I once could? All of these things kept rushing through my mind a lot!

I was feeling depressed. I knew what depression felt like, but this seemed worse than just having a bad or sad day. How would I be able to put into words all my feelings? What does it really mean to be depressed at this time? I would get up, get dressed, have my breakfast, but then I just wanted to sit in fear of my future. It was all so overwhelming. I really hadn't told Valerie all of my feelings because I didn't want her to worry about me. She cared so much and I know it hurt her to see me depressed, but I sluffed some of it off, so she would feel I would be okay and would be my old self again, even though I was wondering if I would ever recover and pull out of this depression and lowliness of feeling I was not worth very much anymore. I also had a thought that maybe Valerie would be better off without me. Should I even be alive? Why did I survive this heart attack? Why didn't God just take me home? Would He really have a purpose for someone with a defective heart? Would He really be able to use me in a weaker state? Who can I help if I cannot lift more than 10-20 pounds? Will I ever be able to lift heavy weights again? I work at a steel company; I have to move heavy steel every day; how is this going to affect my ability to do my job efficiently? How could I share Jesus with anyone when I am wondering if I can be an effective witness of His glory? How can I convincingly share God's love for someone when I feel so unworthy of His love in this weak state? How can I be an effective witness for His kingdom?

So, Pastor Don was here, and I needed to talk to him. I didn't know what to expect. He began by telling me about his experience and feelings when he had his heart attack. He had a much more extensive procedure with open heart surgery, but he understood how debilitating it could be and the feelings that go along with recuperating; learning how to eat differently and listening to what the doctors say, despite how I might feel about it.

He basically gave me the proverbial kick in the butt and told me to stop feeling sorry for myself, do exactly what the doctors told me to do, pray, listen to God and trust Him! His words really hit me like a ton of bricks and made me wake up and stop wallowing in self-pity. That is when my new life started!

Pastor Don's words jerked me out of my "funk." I felt the depression lift off of me after he left and as the day went on. I realized my life was not over and I could still be the husband Valerie deserved, the father James deserved, the leader and mentor of the family and an actual contributor to society and God's kingdom. I felt a surge of love and power from God and the power of the Holy Spirit and a strength I had not felt since I had come home from the hospital! I felt a renewed sense of purpose, encouragement, joy, happiness, peace and an urgency to do everything the doctors were telling me to do, so I can get on with the life God wanted for me!!!

It was later on that day, after thinking about everything I had gone through up until the current moment that I decided to change my attitude, to stop feeling as though I was the only person having to deal with all of this, and most of all, stop allowing the enemy to bring me down to such a low place that I would not be effective in God's kingdom and to those around me! I had a resurgence to create a new life for myself with God's direction and help! I did have a fresh start, so to speak; I beat the widow-maker, because God wanted me here, and I was going to take full advantage of it. I saw it as a wake-up call by God to get down-to-business of taking care of myself, taking medicine for my blood pressure and now for my heart, exercising like I had not been exercising in years, eating in a healthy manner and doing everything I needed to do to prevent another heart attack from ever happening again!

I felt hopeful, re-energized, pumped up, and excited to start the new chapter in my life immediately! Life was going to be good, and God was going to lead me with his grace, mercy, power, might and unconditional love!

The very next day, I got up in the morning and had a joy in my heart about walking with a new vigor and determination. Over the two months of recuperating, I covered a lot of ground walking around my neighborhood, walked a lot of miles and gaining strength and energy with every step. I enjoyed the Southern California weather; it was sunny, bright, a chill would be in the air in the morning because they have some type of winter. It's not the same kind of winter as back near Chicago, but they felt it was winter. My wife and I wouldn't wear a coat when it was 50 degrees outside, but people in Southern California would complain about how cold it was. We would laugh and tell them it was not cold; 10

degrees is cold! We laughed about it a lot with our friends each year. We would tell people, "It's winter!!! It's supposed to be cold!!!" It was always funny to us for people to complain about it being cold in winter – LOL!!!

Well, walking is great, but I eventually became very bored with walking, seeing the same things, on the same streets. Also, I have flat feet, so after building up my stamina to take long aggressive walks, my feet would hurt and it was hard to walk for the rest of the day, and then the next day. I did keep walking, but I needed to find an alternative to walking to get in shape and strengthen my heart.

I talked to my doctor about my new hope and Dr. Steve, who was a cyclist, recommended I start cycling to take pounding off my flat feet. I could gain the health I needed in a new and different way. I had not even thought of cycling as a way to help me improve my health (I had been a wrestler in high school, I loved playing basketball with my Dad, I rode motorcycles, and went off-roading in my Scouts over the years between Elmhurst, IL and California), but I listened to every word Steve was telling me. Steve stated walking on my flat feet was too much. I needed to stop hurting my feet, and his suggestion of taking up cycling intrigued me.

After I left Steve's office, I immediately headed for the Yucaipa Bike Center, a local shop that I knew about in the Uptown District of our city. I really had renewed hope and an excitement that I could hardly contain, even though I was a little nervous and scared at the thought of cycling; however, I knew God would give me the strength, energy and wisdom, so I began my new adventure in this bike shop! It was starting to be exciting for me!!!

I nervously drove to the bike store, because I really didn't know what to expect; I didn't even know what questions I should ask. I definitely did not have an idea of what kind of bike would be right for me to ride. It had been a long time since I rode my banana seat bike as a young boy and my Schwinn as teenager. I just didn't have a clue about the kind of bikes this bike shop sold. As I got closer to the bike store, I became more nervous and anxious, but also excited and scared about it all at the same time. I wanted to get healthy and do something very different from walking, and my doctor made it sound very appealing, along with the fact I wouldn't be hurting my feet by cycling, but I just wasn't sure what it would be like riding a bike around my neighborhood!

It was amazing to walk into the bike store and see all the bicycles. I really didn't know there could be so many different types of bicycles: tall, short, touring, road, mountain, multi-surface riding bikes, etc. I was excited about seeing the bikes but nervous because I didn't know anything about bicycles. They had come a long way since I had ridden bikes when I was young. Again, I was remembering my banana seat bike when I was young and my Schwinn bicycle I had as a teenager with only three speeds. That seemed so long ago, and I never thought I would be at a place of riding a bicycle ever again- not really, at least not as a way to concentrate on my health. My son and I had bikes and would ride around when he was growing up, but the bikes at this store were a lot different than the ones we rode for fun as a family. They were all a lot more sophisticated and expensive and there were a lot more factors that went in to finding the right bike for my height, weight, leg length, etc., etc. All things I did not know anything about and took me years to learn.

I could smell the rubber from the tires of the bikes, and there was an air of exuberance in the shop with everyone being proud of the bicycles and riding as a sport. I stood there and tried to take everything in from the bikes on the floor to the seats, baskets, and everything hanging on the walls. It was in a whole new world!

The vast variety of options was overwhelming, but I quickly found someone to help: I met Eric, the owner of the shop. This is where I began my new journey of cycling and becoming a gear masher, which I will explain later. I spoke to Eric, who was truly knowledgeable, encouraging and helpful about what would be best for me. I told him why I wanted to buy a bike and what I was planning on doing with it: getting healthy so I don't have another heart attack. He showed me different bikes with different gears, different pedals, different seats, and different types of wheels and tires and he explained every single bit of each part of a bicycle, so I would understand what he was talking about. There was a lot to learn about bikes and it was a little overwhelming, but I knew God would direct me to the right bike. I also knew God brought me to this bike store, because Eric is a Christian and I felt very comfortable talking to him once my nerves settled down.

After learning, looking, thinking, praying and listening to all the factors and reasons to find the right bike for me, I finally chose to purchase a hardtail mountain bike with a Rockshox fork with 27 speeds. I learned that a hardtail mountain bike is an all-terrain bike that does not have a rear shock and is equipped with either rigid forks or front suspension. A hardtail is also lighter and cheaper than a full-suspension bike and is a great choice for a beginner rider such as me. The fork I chose on the mountain bike was important because it allowed for more travel at the front of the bike, up and down, as a rider goes downhill on an off-road path. It makes for a better ride on the bike. It also would help the bike perform better and when I was going to ride on rough terrain in the mountain area above the ranger station off of Highway 38 on the way up toward Big Bear, it would make the bouncing more comfortable so it would not jostle the seat, my hands and arms. So, the bicycle I chose was an off-road bike, which is used to ride on dirt and rocky trails. The number of speeds help adjust the gears to aid in climbing up the trails and coming down the trails in a safe manner. I could not believe I was buying a mountain bike because of suffering a heart attack. I was feeling ambitious, nervous, anxious, overwhelmed, uncertain and out of my league. I had a lot to learn about bicycles, but now I was going to learn about

Russell C. Anderson and Valerie N. Anderson

riding like I had never ridden before.

I put a deposit on the bike and paid it off over time. I thought it would take a while to pay it off, but God provided money for the purchase. The day finally came when I could make the final payment and pick up my new bike, bringing it home. I started riding it and becoming familiar with riding in my neighborhood and beyond. This was a lot more fun than walking. I could cover more ground, see more of nature and not hurt my feet. I rode for several weeks without a computer on my bicycle, so I did not know how many miles I had ridden or the average speed of each ride. It was good, but the many miles of riding alone, got to be a bit of a drag. Then one day my new neighbor, Mike Quinlin, rolled a Bianchi road bike out of his garage. He was wearing full cycling attire, and I couldn't help but notice him. He asked me if I wanted to go for a ride. And I said, "You betcha!" He affectionately called his bike, "The Italian."

My first ride with Mike was surprisingly long – it was 25 miles over various roads, including Live Oak Canyon Road, a windy road through a canyon that is narrow and hilly. We had a lot of fun, good discussions and laughs. When we arrived back home, I said, "This is my longest ride, so far." He saw that I had two water bottles and had drunk only half of one. He actually got angry at me. He told me that I should have been drinking a bottle of water for about every 10 miles ridden. Especially, in this area and in this kind of heat. At this time, my tongue literally began to swell in my mouth, due to dehydration. I ran inside my home and guzzled water, because this was a sensation I never had before, and I was hoping guzzling the water would fix it. It did! It hasn't happened since.

Mike and I rode many miles together, and I learned a lot from him. He was a very experienced rider, and he shared with me a lot of his knowledge and experiences with road riding. After a while, he told me that I was getting a lot better with my riding and I could actually keep up with him. I notice that I was losing weight, my blood pressure was lower, my pulse was lower and change was really happening. Hope had returned!

My brother, also named Mike, who is not a rider yet (I'm working on him), asked me a question, "Are you glad now that you had the heart attack?" I had to think about it for a little while, and then I said, "No. I'm never glad I had a heart attack. I wish I could have avoided it, but it was the catalyst into a new life. God made a miracle out of my mess – He's good at that. He can take a mess that we make and turn it into something tremendous for His glory!"

Russell C. Anderson and Valerie N. Anderson

Chapter 6

A Road Bike

One of the problems with being a cyclist, is that it can drain your wallet. There's always one more thing you have to buy. While buying a few accessories for my bike at our local bike shop, Yucaipa Bike Center, I noticed some neat road bikes on the floor. I didn't know anything about road bikes or STI shifters or sizing. So, I basically looked and dreamed.

About this time, back home, my neighbor, Mike Quinlin, told me to take his Bianchi up the street. When I was young, I had an old Schwinn Varsity 10-speed with down-tube shifters, a heavy steel free and heavy steel wheels: a small boat anchor. When I rode the Bianchi up the street, I had never ridden a bike that light, quickly up the street. I asked Mike if his computer was set up on kilometers or miles per hour, and he said, "Miles per hour – you were really going that fast." And I said, "I gotta get me one of these."

During the next trip to the bike shop, I met the head mechanic, Marc Nelison. I told him my riding habits and how fast I was going on a mountain bike, and he told me that I needed to consider a road bike. He pointed me to a Cannondale R500, a good entry-level road bike, yet still out of my price range.

As I spoke to Eric, the owner of the bike shop, he knew at one time that I was a certified welder, and he needed someone to make exercise equipment for martial arts that would require a lot of fabrication. It involved different stations, including a heavy bag. In exchange for helping him make this equipment, I could choose a bike.

So I worked on his project for several weeks, purchasing the materials from my work and welding it in my garage. Upon finishing the equipment, Eric came over to my house and inspected what I had finished. He requested a few small changes, and then I disassembled it and helped him get it to his house. I was very pleased with my work, and I think I did a pretty good job. He said he liked it. I then picked up my first, real, road bike. The Cannondale.

I was trained and taught how to use STI shifters and clipless pedals. Clipless pedals, unlike standard platform pedals lock your feet by way of a plate attached to the bottom of the shoe, to the pedals, so a rider can pull up on the pedals, as well as push down to propel the wheels. This especially helps a rider not use extra energy while pedaling. I hated those clipless pedals at first- I fell quite a few times- but I learned. STI (Shimano Total Integration) shifters are a component introduced in 1990 by Shimano that incorporates the shifters and brakes into one unit. Manual lever shifters are more accurate and quicker but take some learning and getting used to their handling.

Another type of pedals are clip pedals; they have straps on the platform of the pedal and the rider has to reach down to the clip to put the clip around each foot. The rider would also have to reach down to release their foot from the peddle before each stop. I thought these were dangerous, and I saw many riders lose their balance and have a difficult time stopping and even falling.

Clipless pedals only need a twist of the foot to release. Although much easier, I still had to remember to twist my foot. I fell a few times getting used to the twisting motion!

Eventually, I discovered eggbeater pedals, and my neighbor Mike and new friend, Marc, used the eggbeaters, also. Eggbeater pedals look like four-sided cake mixing blades, they are light weight and the rider has four areas to be able to clip in with their shoes, which is easier and faster. They were much better than the original clipless pedals, and I didn't fall as much. I still fell, but only because I had to remember to disengage out of the eggbeaters, as opposed to being "stuck" in the clipless pedals.

Mike and I started riding a lot, and Marc would join us, too! I was basically a student to both of these guys, who were seasoned riders. And, again, I had to buy more "stuff". I guess that's part of the fun.

We road frequently out to the Beaumont and Banning area, here in California, which was anywhere from 20 miles to 50 miles per ride, depending on the routes we took. And since we don't live in Kansas, there are hills – big ones! I had to learn about different cassettes and cranks for my bike and learning to appreciate climbing, to like it, and even enjoy it. I tried to be a spinner; Mike is a spinner, pedaling furiously with a high cadence on a low gear. He would have a cadence of 90 to 95 and even 100. Most riders, in my experience, prefer spinning.

Cadence on a bicycle is like the rider and bike are one vehicle; the rider's heart and lungs are the engine. The legs and feet, pedals, chain and gears are the drive train delivering power to the rear wheel. Some engines (cars or human bodies) will develop more power at higher RPM (Revolutions Per Minute) or HBP (Heartbeats Per Minute), but some are at lower rates. Each rider should learn what the most efficient rate is for the most power at the least amount of energy spent. It takes a lot of time on the bike on different roads with different degrees of difficulty. A heart rate monitor is used to measure and identify where a rider is most comfortable for the most stamina and will make riding much more enjoyable. It helps the rider find their lactic acid threshold as well as their "sweet spot" for riding and climbing.

I tried to be a spinner, but my heart rate would increase too high. Marc had taught me about MHR (Maximum Heart Rate). He taught me how to find my MHR, so I needed to now purchase a heart rate monitor. Marc told me that after I warmed up for about 15 minutes, I was to find a hill that was approximately 3 to 4 percent.

I decided to do what Marc suggest. I found a hill that would work only a few miles from my house - San Timoteo Canyon Road (San Tim). It is actually about a 3 percent climb for about 16 miles. I rode on San Tim after warming up and pushed myself until I felt what I thought MHR felt like, which was a point where I could not grasp a breath of air and I felt like my legs went cold. This is not advisable for everyone! My neighbor, Mike, was with me, because I was told not to find my MHR alone, but to have a riding partner.

I found my MHR was 188 beats per minute (BPM). After finding out this information, I learned to train with 60, 70 and 80 percent of my MHR. In doing so, I found my lactic acid threshold, which was 150 to 160 bpm. This basically means that my engine was running at its most efficient revolutions per minutes (rpm) – I was making energy as fast as I was burning it. Almost a euphoric feeling. Climbing became fun!

I also learned that I am a gear masher, not a spinner. A gear masher uses a higher gear, pedals slower and who's cadence is relatively slow about in the 60's to 70's, depending, of course, on the grade of the hill that needs to be climbed, but the rider pushes and pulls on the pedals very hard. My cadence is approximately

60 to 75 rpm. My legs like it!

One of my personal secrets to climbing well is having a visor on my helmet. It may sound a little strange, but I lower my head a little bit, so the visor prevents me from seeing the top of the climb. For me, on a very difficult climb, if I see how far I have to go, it's intimidating. It takes a little energy away. If I can only see 50 to 75 feet in front of me, I tell myself that I'm going to make it to "that crack in the road", "that mile marker" or "that parked car" – any short-term goal to climb to, rather than looking at the climb as a whole. I'm surprised how many riders I have met that use this same technique.

Now that I had a road bike and was learning how to use it, Mike wanted me to go on some organized rides with him.

Chapter 7

The Tours

My first real organized ride was by myself – well not really. It was the Tour of the Canyons during the Redlands Bicycle Classic in 2003. The Redlands Bicycle Classic is a professional bike race in and around Redlands- the city just west of Yucaipa- that draws professional competitive cyclists from all over the nation and even other parts of the world. The Tour of the Canyons was a public ride that they sponsored on a Saturday, in between the races.

I was nervous! This was the first time I was attempting anything like this by myself. The Tour of the Canyons is approximately a 50-mile ride that winds its way up from Redlands to Beaumont and Banning on a diverse route. I don't recall how many riders there were, but there were more than I had ever seen at one time.

The first hill we were going to climb was Sunset Drive. I had never climbed it before – I had only heard about it. Marc and Mike had given me advice on climbing that I had used on previous rides. They told me to never run at a hill – there is no momentum on a bicycle. You set your pace, your cadence, your heart rate and then you climb. So I did! People were passing me like crazy, going very fast, and then something happened that I did not expect. I slowly reeled them back in and passed most of them. It was awesome! I was feeling very good and confident, until, the Saturn Team blew past me while talking to each other on a hill. I was blown away – those guys were good!

When I crested Sunset Drive and knew I had achieved it, I was so excited that I stopped and called my wife, Valerie. I was so happy, and she was so happy, but I still had a long way to go. So, back to riding.

I made my way up through Beaumont and Banning on familiar roads that I had ridden with Marc and Mike. On the way back toward Redlands, on the return route, which went down San Tim, I had a significant occurrence in my riding adventures. On the way down San Tim, we encountered a strong head wind. I was with four other riders – I didn't even know their names, but one had a Cannondale with a head shock – I thought that was cool. The head wind was so strong, it was everything we could do to maintain 15 miles per hour, downhill. We got into something I had never done before – a pace line. A pace line is where riders ride very close behind each other with their front wheel being only about 10 inches away from the back wheel of the rider in front of them and all of the riders form a pace line. The leader leads until they cannot hold the pace any longer, and slips back alongside the line, to the rear of the line. The next rider is now the leader. I don't particularly like this, because it is difficult to enjoy the scenery.

When it came to being my turn as the leader, I really didn't know what I was doing, but I knew that I could literally feel the riders behind me. A term that riders use for this is "wheel sucking." I tried as hard as I could to hold the pace. I led for quite a while, and it was very taxing. Upon arriving at the Stop and Go Station (SAG) with water, fluid replacement drinks, energy bars, cookies and fruit, a place for the riders, the rider that was directly behind me, came up beside me. He told me, "We sucked your wheel for 5 miles – good job!" I was so ecstatic that someone was impressed with my ability, I said out loud to myself, "I can really do this! Praise God!" It actually felt good to feel the cycling pains everybody else felt.

I continued on – finished the ride and met my wife and son at the finish line in downtown Redlands. There were people at the finish line clanging cow bells and yelling with my wife and son, "Good Job! – You did it!" It was a great accomplishment that taught me a lot about riding and how much I could do. I had certainly come a long way from the guy flat on his back in the ER, getting his heart patched up.

My next organized tour was the 2003 Tour de Palm Springs,

which I rode with Mike. The difference between this ride and the others is that this is a "charity" ride. Mike told me that they don't have a cap on it, so I should expect to see a lot of registered riders. We signed up for the 55-mile ride, and my wife and son, James, went with me. The plan was to stay at my dad's house in Desert Hot Springs, which was only a few miles from the event, saving us a long drive on race day. Valerie and my son, James, were going to overnight with me and attend the event as my cheer squad.

On the morning of the event, Valerie was helping me prepare for the ride. She suddenly turned to me and said, "I'm so proud of you! Right now, two years ago, you were in a hospital bed recovering from a heart attack and now you're riding the Tour de Palm Springs!" It sure helps to have someone this good in your corner.

We got ready and met Mike near the flag pole at the Palm Springs High School, where the Tour was going to begin. Mike and I got our registration numbers to pin to our jerseys and put on our bikes and proceeded over to the other side of the school where all of the 55-mile riders were gathering. Mike made sure we both had GU (pronounced goo), which is an energy gel that you squeeze into your mouth, about five minutes before you begin climbing a big hill or when you begin to feel that you're running out of energy.

He also taught me about tandem cyclists. He told me that during a ride, sometimes a tandem bike with pass you and riders will dive in behind it, to draft off of the tandem bike. A tandem bike has about 50 percent more weight, but twice the riders, and a good tandem team will pass a lot of riders. He encouraged me to watch for them.

The ride started around 7:00 a.m. with approximately 4,600 riders – WOW! We saw bikes from Wal-Mart to every major bike manufacturer in the world, from a bike that might cost $70 to a more expensive, elite road bike that could cost $5,000. In the beginning of the ride, it was very crowded, and I felt like I was riding in a crowded elevator but, just as Mike had told me, the riders spread out as the race went on and we soon had elbow room.

There are no big hills in this ride – just long slow hills of about 2 to 3 percent, one grinder about 18 miles into the ride and a lot of flat, fast riding. Mike and I had a lot of fun and a lot of conversations along the way. Then, low and behold, a tandem flew by us with about two riders behind it. Mike and I jumped on the train, and we were passing large groups of riders. I was feeling exceptionally energetic, and after about a mile or so, I pulled out and passed the tandem. Of course, I couldn't hold that pace for too long, Mike caught up and said, "You're not supposed to pass the tandem!" I said, "I was just feeling exceptionally strong – it was a lot of fun!"

The ride was well maintained, had good SAGs, and it was an overall tremendous experience. There were a few crashes, but we did not see any; we just heard about them at the end of the ride after we got back to the starting point. Valerie and James were there waiting for my arrival and cheered when they saw me walking my bike toward the flag pole. My average on the ride was 16.5 miles per hour, which is good but not great, yet I was happy with that pace. Mike left to go home and Valerie, James and I went to the Blue Coyote Café in Palm Springs to have a celebratory lunch. At lunch, I had my first experience of feeling severe cramping in my thighs. After lunch, we headed home so I could rest, rest, rest!

At this time, in 2003, I started doing my morning rides, Mondays through Fridays, about 3 to 4 weekdays and then Saturdays, I would typically go on a longer ride. During the week, I would get up around 6:00 a.m. and ride for about 8 to 10 miles. After a little while, Mike joined me on these morning rides. We would ride a fairly flat route for this area, and I found it gave me energy for the day.

In Southern California, we can ride all year long. Of course, it is much colder during the winter months of January, February and March. December can be cold, but it is still in the 40's and 50's. April can be chilly, but, again, it is usually in the 40's and 50's in the mornings. During January, February and March, it is colder, not Chicago cold, but cold for this area. I've seen it as low as 25 degrees where we live, and I won't ride when it is that cold. In my earlier days of riding, 2003, 2004, and 2005, I would go out in 30 plus degree weather – of course, bundled up. Mike would be just as bundled up, but sometimes Mike did not want to ride when it was that cold. In the latter years of my morning rides, the cold stopped being as fun! Or, maybe I just got smarter!

Around 2006, I discovered that longer rides in the morning, about three days a week, was more beneficial to training. I started getting up around 4:45 a.m., so I could start riding around 5:00 a.m., preparing my bottles and bike the night before. I increased my mileage to 15-20 miles each morning. My routes got a little longer and a little more interesting. I cannot emphasize enough the importance of good lights, especially wearing one on the helmet. There have been many times during my morning rides where people are going to work or school, they're in a hurry and do not stop at stop signs or stop lights. With the helmet light, I can shine it toward the driver, to ensure they see me. I also have a bike-mounted headlight and rear blinking lights mounted on the bike. I have also discovered that people driving in the morning were more patient than people coming home in the evening. I used to ride in the evening, but people had already been at work and on the freeway and were a little frustrated, making riding a little more dangerous – at least in our area. The morning rides are a great way to start my day.

I also started seeing interesting things and animals on my morning rides. I have seen many coyotes, a lot of rabbits, a few bobcats, emus, zebras, etc. As you guessed, we live in a more rural area. On one particular Thanksgiving morning, I went on my EMT (Earn My Turkey) ride. While riding down Grape Street, a side street off of Bryant Street, I reached the point where I turned around to go to another neighborhood. When I turned around, I was looking at a mountain lion, approximately 400 feet from me on the road. We both stopped and looked at each other for about 15 seconds. I knew I could not try to get away, because I was on a hill and I could just become prey. I thought two things instantly – I hope you're full, and I've got to start carrying a camera, because no one's going to believe me! Luckily for me, he must have already had his breakfast, because he trotted off into the weeds. Now I carry a camera on every ride, but I haven't seen him since.

We live right below the mountain town of Oak Glen. The Oak Glen loop, as it is called, is a difficult climbing ride. From my driveway, around the loop and back to my driveway is only 20 miles, but there is 2,500 feet of climbing. We would do this ride, occasionally, on Saturdays, and of course, add some extra miles.

In 2004, I bought a mountain bike, which added new rides to my routine. I bought a Specialized Rock Hopper – a full-suspension bike – something new to learn. Mike, Marc and I would do a lot of single-track riding, but I was predominantly a roadie. During this year, I participated in my second Tour de Palm Springs.

For the 2004 Tour de Palm Springs, I rode with Mike again. My wife, son and I went to Palm Springs the night before the ride and participated in their spaghetti dinner for the riders to carb load. The Honorary Cyclist was Huell Howser, whom we got to meet. Huell was a Southern California celebrity who had a weekly TV show called California's Gold, that celebrated events and locales throughout the state. He rode in the Tour the next day. He was professional and humorous as an Honorary Cyclist. He asked me what ride I was doing, and I told him the 55-miler, and he stated that he was only doing the 25-mile ride.

We met Mike again at the flag pole of the Palm Springs High School, and the route was basically the same as the previous year, except there were a lot more riders – around 8,000, give or take a few. This ride wasn't very eventful, and I held the same average as the previous Tour, 16.5 miles per hour. After the ride, Valerie, James and I went to the Blue Coyote Café in Palm Springs again, which we deemed our traditional restaurant for our celebratory lunches after every Tour de Palm Springs. In all, I rode in ten Tour De Palm Springs', one of which was the 100-mile ride.

In 2005, I gave my Cannondale road bike to my son, James, after I had upgraded everything on the bike, except for the fork and the frame. Two things I want to mention here: 1) The Cannondale was my first official road bike and I put 12,000 miles on it; I have no complaints. And, 2) I'm very proud of my son. After he received the bike in December of 2005 for Christmas, James wanted to start riding with me. I had replaced the Cannondale with a Trek 2200 road bike, so we went out on a couple of local rides together, and he did well. He then told me he wanted to do the Tour de Palm Springs with me. I warned him that it would be a serious ride, a significant amount of miles, and a lot of riders. He said he still wanted to ride it with me. And I said, "Okay, let's do it!"

About 20 miles into the ride, while filtering through the crowd, a rider came up next to James and did not say, "On your left" as he was passing James. They tangled, and in my mirror, I saw wheels and pedals in the air. James was scraped up a bit, had a couple of bruises, and was a little shaken up. After a few moments to gather his senses, he said he wanted to continue and finish the ride! I was amazed and proud! I think that if that was my first long ride, I would have stopped. I'm very pleased that James chose to finish the ride, and we did it together. It was a great moment in my life!

2005 was the year I rode the most miles, 5,413. Not bad, for working full time at a steel plant! I haven't ridden that many miles that many miles again, because I found myself trying to put miles on my bikes every chance I could and, by December of that year, I was almost sick of riding. I love cycling and how it has redeemed my health, so I didn't want to burn out by overriding.

For Thanksgiving of that year, Valerie and I went to Missouri to visit her Mom. I knew that they would be talking crafts, crafts, crafts, family, and crafts – so I rented a bike from a shop in Joplin, MO. It was a Trek 1000, an entry-level road bike. I was grateful that they were willing to rent it to me. Since I had planned on doing this, I had sent my helmet and riding equipment ahead. Upon picking up the bike and after spending that day with

Valerie's mom, I went on three long rides while we were there through Thanksgiving. On one of the rides, I rode from my mother-in-law's house to Fairland, Oklahoma. The roads were predominantly flat with a few grinders, but no big hills. It was extremely beautiful country with a lot of trees and scenery, but I missed the big hills of California. I called Valerie when I got to Oklahoma and she could not believe that I had ridden to another state! The entire ride was 70 miles long.

A saying that I heard over the years, is that "Smooth seas never made a good sailor." I adapted that to riding and said, "Smooth, flat roads never made a good well-rounded rider." A good rider needs to know how to ride steep hills, ride steep descents, watch out for road hazards, and especially, traffic. Something else, however, that I learned in Missouri about flat roads is that flat roads are not as easy as I thought. Since there are no big hills, there are no big down hills — you pedal all the time. If you stop pedaling, you stop! I have a new respect for long distance riding on flatter roads, but I still long for the hills. Since 2005, my annual numbers have been lower, coming in at around 4,000 miles per year.

Valerie and James rode in a Tour de Palm Springs in 2012 with our riding group, Ride Yourself Fit (RYF), a cycling club in Redlands, CA, which is headed up by our former doctor, Dr. Steven Wilson. This was quite an accomplishment for Valerie, as she had not ridden in over a year and a half. She regretted the ride at first, because the start of the ride was a gradual incline for about three or so miles. She almost quit because it was difficult for her, but she kept going and made it to the top of the climb, turned right onto the street that was part of the route and enjoyed a wonderful downhill.

I rode it with her, even though she was afraid I would get bored, but I told her that I did not want to miss riding with her in her first Tour. It was exciting to see her ride and having fun. When she passed other riders, she cheerfully said, "On the left" and giggled each time. She was riding the Trek Navigator I had bought for her. It was fun for her to ride, but she had a hard time starting and stopping if she wasn't by a curb. So, as she was riding, she would loudly let people know she was there, because she would not have been able to stop well and was afraid of falling over. I saw her laughing and waving her arms for people to get out of the way, which scared me to death a few times, and I was shaking my head a lot.

All of us finished the ride at 12.5 miles, and there was a cheering section, at the end of the ride with a lot of RYF riders and others. Valerie was almost in tears because she couldn't believe she finished the ride and had never been cheered for in such a way in her life. I was so proud of her! I told her that I would do it all over again, any time! She did discover, though, why riders wear the padded bike shorts, which she did not have at the time, because she dealt with a lot of soreness over the next four or five days.

THE HEART ATTACK THAT SAVED MY LIFE

Over the years, I did nine 55-mile Tour de Palm Springs rides and one century Tour de Palm Springs. Eventually, it just got too crowded, which took some of the fun out of it. I then decided to look at other century rides in Southern California, including the Shadow Tour Stagecoach Century Ride out of Ocotillo, California. I also rode in the Solvang Prelude, and the Solvang Century with my riding buddy, Scott.

I want to tell you about Scott. I started riding with him about 8 years ago. He is well over six feet tall. He's a jogger, cyclist and competitive swimmer. He lives close by and we have been on many rides together. Scott's an excellent climber, and I have watched his back wheel going up many hills. He is a better climber than I was, and over the years, I improved by following him and trying to catch him on the hills. My competitive nature had to get to a place where I could beat him on a climb. It was an accomplishment to me when I finally beat him to the top of Sunset. We still ride together, on occasion and have a lot of laughs and good conversation amongst the miles. He is a great friend!

Another health issue I had to address was a whiplash that I received while riding a motorcycle in my teens. My 6th and 7th vertebrae are sitting on top of each other and, according to the doctors, they are fusing together. This causes my hands to frequently go numb on rides. I tried using carbon forks and carbon handlebars, but they helped very little. Steve had an old Trek that had a Paris Roubaix fork. It is a suspension fork designed for the Paris Roubaix Race that provided a one-inch travel. The Paris Roubaix Race is the oldest race, which began in 1896 and is a one-day professional men's bicycle road race in northern France, starting north of Paris and finishing in Roubaix at the border with Belgium. After I saw this fork, I thought it would help my neck, so I searched online and found one for my bike. Unfortunately, it only has a one-inch steerer – most current road bikes have a one and one-eighth steerer. I had to have an adapter specially made at a bike shop and have the fork mounted on the bike. This took a lot of work on their part, but they were able to do it and I was extremely thankful to them for their extra effort. This reduces some of the shock to my neck on bumpy roads, and the numbness in my hands has decreased.

In 2008 I considered buying a recumbent bike, after having heard so many good things about them. I took one for a test ride, but found that climbing inclines wasn't as fun as it is on a regular bike. A recumbent is a bicycle that places the rider in a laid-back reclining position. The weight of the rider is not over the pedals. There are some riders that can climb on recumbents, but I am not one of them. After I test rode the recumbent, I brought it back to Yucaipa Bike Center. That was when I spotted the Felt Dispatch Single Speed. I have never ridden one, so I thought, "Why not?" I took it for a test ride! To my surprise, not only did I like it – I loved it! Being a gear masher, it fit my legs well. So I bought it and started putting miles on it!

Chapter 8

The Dingers

My doctor, Steve, challenged me in 2008 to participate in the organized cycling event, the Ride Around The Bear. This is a road ride that leaves from Sylvan Park in Redlands, California to climb up into the towering San Bernardino Mountains and then back down. The race heads up Highway 330 up through Running Springs, then up to Big Bear, then to Highway 38, over Onyx Summit and then back down to Sylvan Park in Redlands. It is 101 miles and 9,500 feet of climbing. The thought of going on the ride was very intimidating to me. However, I accepted the challenge and began training.

I chose to use my Trek 2200 to train for this event. My training included riding from my home, down through

Redlands, Loma Linda, San Bernardino, going along the Santa Ana River Trail, out to Riverside and Norco and back to my house. The challenge in this is that the course is about 80 miles long and most of the climbing comes after the 60 mile mark. I had to make sure that I could climb late into the ride. I have learned a great deal from my friends and fellow riders about budgeting my energy – not hammering up hills early on in a ride, but remembering that at the 40 or 50 mile mark, I still have 1,500 feet of climbing coming up around the 60 mile mark.

Another training ride is called the D.O.G. – Double Oak Glen, which consists of riding over to 5th Street and Oak Glen Road in Yucaipa, riding up Oak Glen Road, around the top of the town of Oak Glen, back down the other side of the town and to Wildwood Canyon Road and Bryant Street. I then ride on Bryant Street back to Oak Glen Road and climb around Oak Glen again. The total ride is 42 miles long and consists of 5,100 feet of climbing. Not many riders will do this ride with me – I wonder why? Sometimes, it hurts!

Doing a ride similar to the Ride Around The Bear, requires stamina, knowing how to recover on the bike and, of course, having good equipment. Equipment matters! This is a serious ride! I trained for approximately two months for this ride. There is a cap to the number of riders, which is 400 riders, which sounds like a lot, but it's really not. Some rides have 2,000-3,000 riders and the Tour de Palm Springs has around 10,000. So, 400 riders is a much safer number, especially riding up the mountain roads. Prior to this ride, I was also power-fitted to my Trek 2200 by a professional rider, Jim.

Power fitting is more accurate than simply taking measurements to find out what frame size would be correct for your body. That measurement is only a good ballpark figure, but power fitting entails riding your bike on a trainer until you are tired and finding out where you hurt and where how much of your weight is located on each wheel. Jim discovered that since I am very muscular in my upper body, I had too much weight on my front wheel, and not enough over the pedals. A simple fix of a much taller handle bar stem took 10.5 pounds off of my front wheel and over my pedals. This made my climbing more efficient. Jim told me that since I am built more like a weight lifter than a cyclist, I will climb long and I will climb strong but I will not climb fast. He told me that I had to accept that fact if I was going to do long rides with a lot of climbing. If I hammer up a hill to stay with a smaller, lighter rider, I would burn my batteries up on that hill and since we live in the hills, there would be another hill after that to climb. So, I adjusted my style of riding,

59

using my gears and letting my heart-rate govern my speed. Climbing now became even more fun for me.

My first Ride Around The Bear went very well. I rode it with Steve and other cycling friends, even though I could not maintain their speed. Highway 330, for me, is the hardest part of the ride. It's about 8 percent incline for about 8 miles. The ride took me into Running Springs and around the back side of Big Bear Lake, and then up Highway 38 to Onyx Summit. At Onyx Summit, another rider and I took commemorative pictures (like the one on the front cover) and continued down toward Redlands. On the way down the back side, there is a place I call the "Dirty Trick" which is because after going downhill for about 7 miles, my legs are cold, and my heart rate is in the 70's, and I think I'm done climbing.

A few miles short of arriving at Angeles Oaks, there is a mile of 9 percent climbing. My legs locked up for I have a problem with cramping. Over the years, this has occurred on long rides with a significant amount of climbing. I kind of knew this would happen because Steve had been working on this problem with me over the years, advising me about sodium, magnesium, potassium and drinking enough water. Valerie told me about using up salt in the body when sweating a lot and how she had to take salt tablets and drink almost a gallon of water while eating salty crackers when she became dehydrated and drained when backpacking in Wisconsin with the Girl Scouts. Walking it out and stretching would help my legs minimally. I remembered how I would have salt lines on my bike shorts after long, hot, strenuous rides. So, I had a few packets of salt with me; I just poured the salt in my mouth and drank my electrolyte water, which I carried on every ride. Within a few minutes, my legs stopped cramping and I was back on my bike riding toward the finish.

After arriving in Angeles Oaks, it is a blitz after the SAG stop into Redlands – all downhill. Riders have to be careful, because the road is quite windy at times. Valerie was waiting for me at the finish line, cheering me on and yelling, "Good job" and clanging a cow bell. I was so pleased that I completed the ride – the training helped tremendously.

I rode my second Ride Around The Bear in 2010, on the same bike, my Trek 2200, and the ride went pretty much the same way as the first one. I rode it again with Steve and my cycling friends. Again, Valerie met me at the end of the ride, and I must say, The Orange County Wheelmen do a great job putting on this ride. Very few incidences or crashes occur and the route is well marked, the SAG stops are well stocked and help is always close by for the riders. A lot of care is taken to help the riders succeed.

Steve was very impressed with my accomplishment, and on a future ride to the beach with Ride Yourself Fit, he asked me to give my testimony about my heart attack, recovery, cycling and improved health. I was honored and blessed to give my testimony, and I hope I was an encouragement to people struggling with health problems.

In 2010, I also did a century ride with a close friend, Glenn Ousley. This man was such a strong rider, he could climb Oak Glen in his big ring. He and I decided to do a century ride starting at Yucaipa Bike Center, heading along various roads to Norco and then heading back up to the far end of Banning and back to the bike shop. This ride was 112 miles long and had 4,000 feet of climbing. When we returned, I was exhausted, but Glenn went to work at the bike shop. We called our ride the RG Century Plus (Russ and Glenn).

We were able to do our ride the next year, our last year. We planned on doing the ride again but, unfortunately, Glenn became very sick and eventually passed away. I miss him a lot. He was a great rider, a great friend and a tremendous person who touched a lot of lives in this community.

THE HEART ATTACK THAT SAVED MY LIFE

In 2012, I decided to get stupid. My neighbor, Mike and I, had a fun phrase between each other. We would be out on a ride and spot a hill and say, "Let's get stupid and try and climb that." Remember, some of us cyclists are not very bright – we will ride to another town to climb a hill and ride back. It's a strange form of fun! I decided that the first two Ride Around The Bear rides didn't hurt enough. So, I wanted to find out if I could do the ride on my single speed. I actually feel that God challenged me to do it!

My Felt Single Speed came with a 36 crank ring and a 16 cog and through White Industries, I bought a 22 tooth freewheel cog, and I changed my front ring to a 32 and started training. I also purchased strong wheels by Cane Creek that has the threaded part of the spoke in the hub, so there is no bend in the spoke – they are straight pulls. They are exceptional wheels and very strong. I bought these, because in training, I learned that a single speed creates a great amount of torque, and I kept breaking spokes. After many thousands of miles, and many thousands of feet of climbing, I still have the same spokes and the same wheels on my Felt!

I did the same training on this bike that I did on the Trek 2200. Being as my riding style is more of a gear masher than a spinner, my legs like the hard cranking of the single speed. My neighbor, Mike, made me promise him that if I felt any pain in my knees, I would take a SAG ride down to the finish. H was not favor of me doing the Ride Around The Bear on my single speed. I said that I would – I made him the promise.

My wife encouraged me through all of my training and kept saying, "I know you can do it!" In all honesty, I wasn't sure that I could. I guess that's why it was a challenge.

We started the ride at Sylvan Park in Redlands, Steve and other riders with RYF were at the park. We left early, because it is a long day. The route was a little different going up Highway 38 to Green Spot – this is a decent climb in itself – a good warm up. We made our way over the base of Highway 330, and this is where I got off the bike and turned my wheel around to the climbing gear, the 22 cog. I looked up the road; it looked daunting. I remembered all of the lessons that I had learned over the years from Marc and Mike about climbing and started up the mountain.

To me, Highway 330 is the hardest part of the route. As I said before, 8 percent for a long time. I set my cadence, my breathing and my heart rate and maintained my pace of around 150 beats per minutes (bpm). What a gorgeous ride - mountains, trees, tremendous views of the valley, and the weather was perfect!

When I reached the first SAG stop, I was excited and relieved. I also knew to not stop for too long, because I did not want my legs to get cold – ten minutes tops. I filled my bottles, ate a banana and some peanut butter, stretched and got back on the bike. I started climbing again toward Running Springs. I began feeling some cramping at the second SAG stop.

One problem that I had leading up to my heart attack is high blood pressure, so my doctor put me on a low sodium diet to coincide with the medication to lower my blood pressure. The problem with this, once I started riding very strenuously, I would sweat a lot and sweat out the salt that was in my body. This, I discovered, contributed to the cramping in my legs. So, something I learned over the years regarding cramping, that works for me, but I do not recommend to everyone, is that I would bring salt packets from fast food restaurants with me on the rides. When I felt the cramps starting, I would sprinkle about half of a packet of salt onto my tongue. This helped a lot, because for me, it was replenishing the salt I was sweating out. I made sure to discuss everything that I would test to get rid of my cramps with my doctor! My cramping went away and I continued on the ride.

Being as there are only approximately 400 riders,

there are times during the ride when I would not see any other rider for several miles. This was a wonderful alone time amongst nature. I would also be thanking God for strengthening me for the challenge, and of course, praying for safety.

When I reached Big Bear, I had a feeling of excitement and accomplishment and took a picture by the city's sign. I continued riding around the north shore of the lake to a turn that crossed the lake to Highway 38. This led to the climb to Onyx Summit, the highest point of the ride. I have done this portion of the route before, having ridden in this organized ride two times in the past. This usually is not the hardest part of the ride, because it is about a 4 percent grade for approximately 7 miles. Not a big climb, but after almost 7,500 feet of climbing, it can be difficult. Of course, unlike the other times, I had a small tail wind. I would have thought this would be good, but when you are riding around 7 miles per hour on a climb, and the wind is blowing around 7 miles per hour, the air is dead – I was baking. Many riders were complaining about the same thing, and we were praying for a small head wind to cool us off. I also must note that during the entire ride I got strange looks from riders when they did not see a cassette on my back wheel. They would say, "You're doing this on a single speed? Are you nuts?" And I said, "Could be!"

During the time climbing to Onyx Summit, I was very close to obtaining a SAG ride to the finish line. The heat and lack of being able to cool off, was draining my energy. At one point in a turn out, a man in a SAG vehicle asked me if I wanted a ride down – I thought about it. However, I knew that if I took the ride, I could not say that I climbed Big Bear on a single speed. So, I toughed it out and kept going!

I can't tell you the great feeling I had when I rounded the corner and saw the Onyx Summit sign. My energy came back and I felt overwhelmed that I was going to make it to the end. Upon reaching the sign, of course, I had someone take my picture next to the sign. I then went to the SAG stop and refilled my bottles again, aged a little bit and started the long trip down the mountain. Now the ride became cold, because after sweating in the heat, the wind was cooling me off.

I remembered that the "Dirty Trick" was coming in about 6 or 7 miles. Around 6 miles into the descent, I started spinning my pedals vigorously, trying to get my heart rate up and warming up my legs. Unfortunately, this did not work. As soon as I hit the "Dirty Trick", the 9 percent climb, my legs locked up. Even though this climb is only about one mile long, the cramping was so bad that

I had to get off of the bike. I walked the bike for about a quarter of a mile. When I did this on my Trek 2200, a 27-speed bike, I had what I like to refer to as a "dinner plate" on the back wheel – a 34-tooth cog. I would simply shift into this and keep my legs spinning. It is really the best thing to do when you begin cramping – ride slowly through it. I could not do this on a single speed.

After walking the short distance, which uses different muscles than cycling, the cramps eased, and I got back on the bike and finished the short climb. I then continued down the mountain to Angeles Oaks, the last SAG stop. This is where I heard one of my favorite compliments. At each SAG, sometimes, there are volunteers who will hold a rider's bike while they refill their bottles and get snacks. When a volunteer held my bike, he looked down at the gearing and he said, "You need your head examined!" I laughed!

After filling my bottles and getting something to eat, I continued down the mountain – it was all downhill from there. It was extremely fast and windy, and I remember yelling, "Praise God – I did it, I did it, I did it!!!"

I arrived at Sylvan Park, saw Valerie cheering for me and taking pictures. I actually felt pretty good. I saw a lot of my riding friends and we shared our stories about the ride. I heard Valerie bragging about me and telling any rider she could that I had done the ride on a single speed. She found out that there was one rider who did it on a recumbent, which is also a tremendous feat in itself. We grabbed something to eat and headed home for a good night's sleep.

Steve was proud of my accomplishment, and he posted a picture on the RYF website telling of my success. Mike asked me about the ride, and I told him that my knees never hurt, I wasn't in any danger, there weren't any incidences or near misses, and I finished the ride! Scott and Mike were both very impressed with the ride I had completed. Scott told me he didn't think he could do it, and I said, "You're a better climber than me – you could do it!" Mike said he would only do it if they would close the road to cars.

I don't plan on trying that ride again on a single speed. I'm a little older and a little more concerned about my legs not being able to handle the difficulty of that climb in one gear. It's a bad thing to be wrong about. I still ride a lot and do a lot of climbing, but I'm a little more aware of my body's limitations.

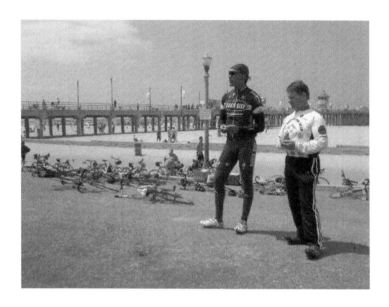

At the beach, giving my testimony to our Ride Yourself Fit group at the end of the first leg of a Santa Ana River Train Ride. Dr. Steven Wilson is on the left.

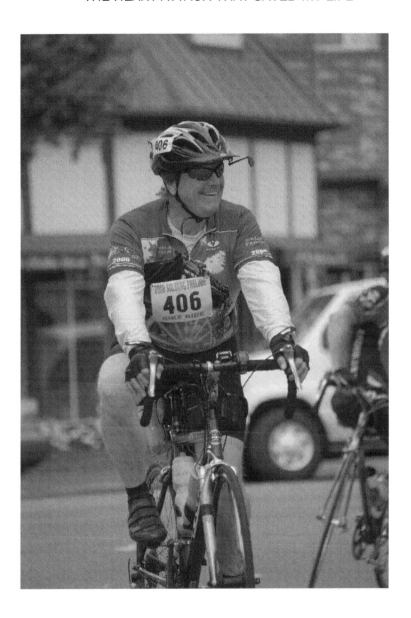

The Solvang Prelude on my Trek 2200!

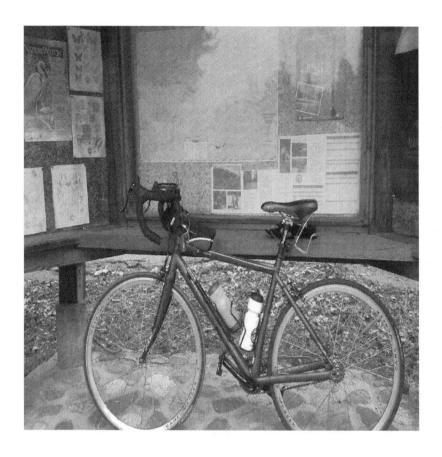

My Felt Dispatch Single Speed at the top of Oak Glen during a training ride!

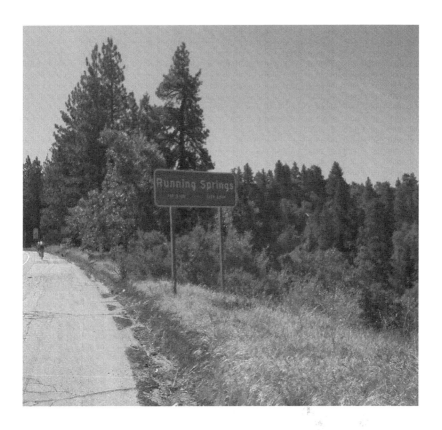

Small victory – arriving in Running Springs during the Ride
Around The Bear!

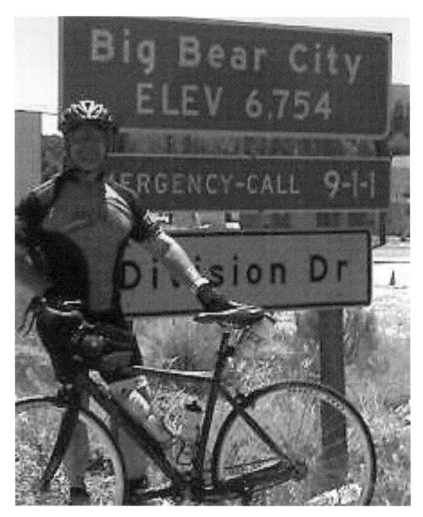

Arrived in Big Bear City – what a beautiful and difficult climb!

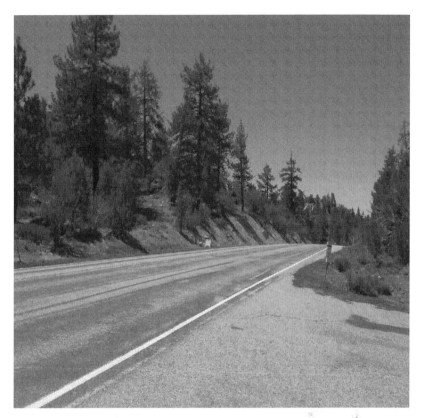

The Climb to Onyx Summit during the Ride Around The Bear!

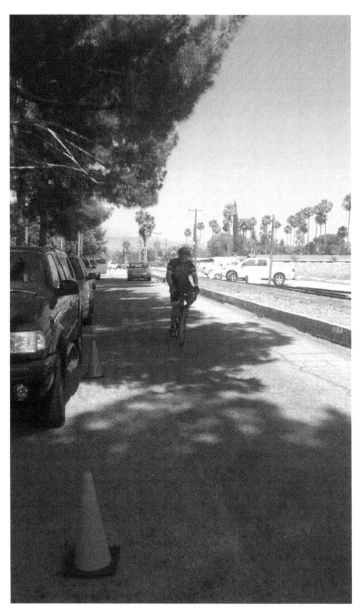

Arriving back at Sylvan Park after completing The Ride Around The Bear! Valerie was cheering me on and took the picture.

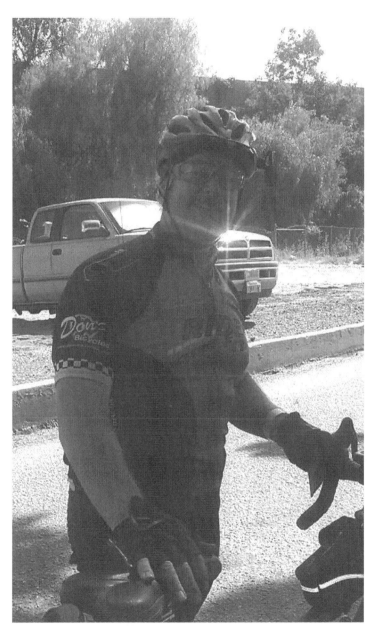

Wow – I did it!! Praise God!!! Thank you, Valerie, for your support!!!

Russell C. Anderson and Valerie N. Anderson

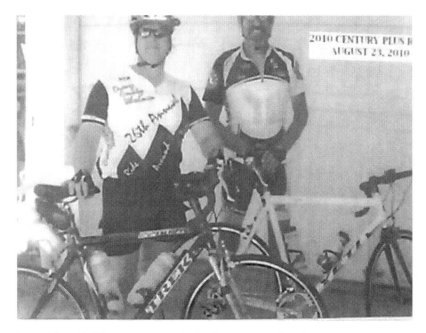

Myself and Glenn on our RG Century Ride, August 23, 2010!

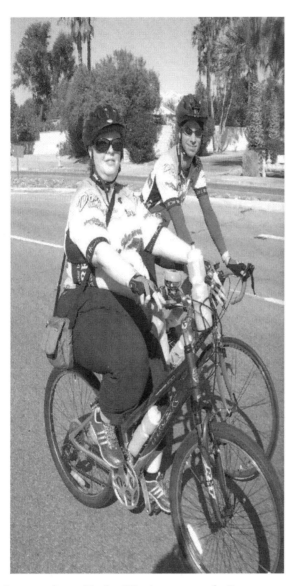

Valerie on her Trek Navigator and James on the Cannondale during the 2012 Tour de Palm Springs. Since this picture, Valerie has lost over 75 pounds!

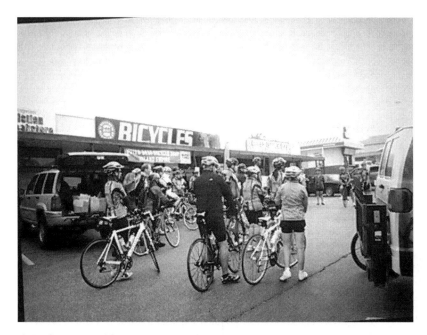

A Ride Yourself Fit (RYF) Ride leaving from Yucaipa Bike Center!

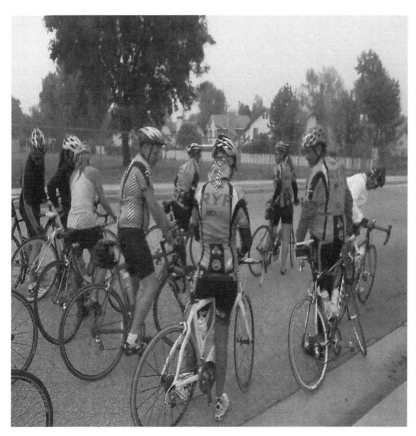

Ride Yourself Fit (RYF) Cycling Club members!

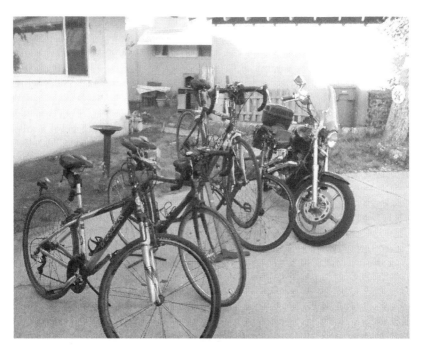

I spend a lot of time on two wheels!

Chapter 9

What I've Learned

I called this book, "The Heart Attack That Saved My Life", because it saved my life in so many ways. It obviously brought to my attention a health scare – my poor cardiovascular health, my lack of confidence, and my lack of determination. I started riding, obviously for health reasons, but it became so much more. There is a saying that I learned: there is nothing glorious about hills; they just hurt. However, I believe that saying is completely wrong. When I get to the top of a hill that I should not be able to climb, I feel good; it is glorious! The comradery between riders is tremendous. When I started feeling cycling pains and not heart pains, they were very welcomed. That may not make sense to some, but I think to athletes it will.

I don't know what the Lord has in store for me in the miles ahead, but praise God, I will give Him the glory!

Will Rogers said, "Even if you're on the right track, you'll get run over if you just sit there." I do know that I will not always be able to work as I work now, or ride as I ride now – there will be a day when I wish I could, but I won't be able to. So, while I can – I will!

Enjoy your adventure!

WHAT??? THERE'S MORE.....

Chapter 10

Oh Crap! I Really Didn't See That One Coming!

In the evening of August 3, 2018, I was outside around 10:30 p.m. It was a Friday night, and I needed to take some sound equipment out of my truck and put it in the garage, so I would have room to put my drums in the truck for practice the next day with my band.

I was moving two main speakers from the truck into the garage. I had backed the truck up to the garage, so it was not a long distance to carry the equipment, but it was far enough for what would happen next.

I took two heavy speakers out of the truck and set them individually on the ground. I then lifted both of them (each weighing about 55 lbs.); one in each hand. As I lifted them to walk into the garage, I felt a twinge in my chest. I had felt this before, but I set the speakers down immediately and tried again. The twinge happened again! I got the speakers into the garage, despite the twinge, closed the garage door and locked up the truck, because I knew what was happening.

I went inside after locking everything up and took an aspirin and my blood pressure medicine. Neither helped change the feeling in my chest I was having. I went and sat down on my side of the bed and sat quietly. Valerie was still awake, turned over and ask me, "What's wrong?" I told her, "I'm having a heart attack."

Valerie immediately got up, got dressed and whisked me out the front door to drive me safely and expediently fast to Redlands Community Hospital to the Emergency Room. Yes, we did think about calling the ambulance, but we decided, again, to have Valerie drive me. I think we actually arrived at the hospital faster than if we had waited for the ambulance, but of course, we will never know.

I sat down in the waiting room, and Valerie quickly

got up to the admission window. She told the nurse that I had a heart attack in 2001 and, "He is having another heart attack right now!" The nurse immediately let staff know that I was there, having a heart attack, at which time, the door opened to the back area and I was rushed to a bed to begin tests.

Valerie had to stay at the window to make sure they had our insurance, my name, and all the other information they must have to admit someone into the hospital. Then, a nurse came to the window and stated that Valerie had to come back there quickly to where I was, because there is an urgent matter. She handled it like a trooper and stayed calm.

When she got back to where I was, she was greeted by the head of the transport ambulance, as well as an entire team; doctors, nurses, someone taking my blood, someone else giving me medication, two or three ambulance staff. All greeted her very kindly and professionally and began to explain what was happening with me.

She was told, as I had been told when the EKG was being done, that there was a blurp on the EKG and they needed to rush me to Loma Linda University Medical Center (LLUMC) immediately. They told her that I did have a heart attack and the concern about what they saw on the EKG was so great that they needed to rush me full speed with sirens to LLUMC for immediate surgery. She asked where the emergency room was located at Loma Linda, they told her, she came over and gave me a kiss, told me it was going to be okay and that she loved me; she left immediately to meet the ambulance at the other hospital.

The news was shocking to both of us, because I felt so good; unlike how I felt during my first heart attack. I was awake, talking and felt that I could jump off the gurney and go home. But of course, that was not going to happen, and we found out later why it was not going to happen.

The ambulance was already there when she pulled into a parking place, and she saw me being wheeled into the next emergency room at LLUMC. The guard at the desk immediately directed her which direction to go to see me, and she arrived to meet a new set of team members for my case. The doctor spoke to her immediately and told her that they were going to take me in for surgery immediately to the Cath Lab. She gave me another kiss, said she loved me, and they whisked me away for surgery within 20 minutes of my arrival. Valerie had to stay back to help the nurse get me checked into this hospital. This part of the process was very stressful for Valerie, because she saw me being rolled away by a team of doctors and nurses and she did not know where I was and how to see me.

After she completed getting me checked into the hospital, a very kind nurse helped Valerie find where I was having the surgery (after not knowing himself and calling down to the emergency area to find out exactly where I was) and where she could wait for me to get out of surgery.

The surgery was over and by 3:00 a.m. on Saturday, August 4, 2018, I had been to two emergency rooms, been diagnosed, had surgery and was in my room in the Cardiac ICU Unit of Loma Linda University Medical Center. It was a whirlwind of events that I never saw coming!

I had to stay in the hospital until Monday, August 6th, despite the doctors telling me every day I was going to go home the same day or the next day. As I stayed in the hospital, God kept doing things over and over and let me and my wife know that he was with us all the time and was watching out for us!

When I saw the doctors after my surgery, later in the morning of August 4th, I learned things about my heart attack that I could not have imagined. My cardiologist told me that I had a massive heart attack on the LAD, which is the largest artery of the heart and is called "The Widow Maker." He and a team of doctors, and interns (since Loma Linda is a teaching hospital) told me that my heart attack was in the same artery as my first heart attack. He also told me they had cleaned out the old stent that was in the LAD and added a new one inside the old one that was longer, which made it go beyond both ends of the first one and my cardiac function was 25-30, which the normal is around 50. He also told me that I had grown two bypasses due to my athletic cycling because my body needed more oxygen and if that had not happened, I would have died in my garage.

All of this was shocking to Valerie and I, because when I had the first heart attack, we were not told which artery, and we were not told my cardiac function. Valerie began to cry because she was in shock with all the news and realized that God kept me alive by His grace. I was also in shock at all the news and a little angry that we did not get all this information for my first heart attack; of course, it had been 17 and a half years earlier and a lot of things had changed in cardiac knowledge and care since then. Technically, I beat the "Widow Maker" TWICE!

My doctor could not quite explain why the heart attack happened, except to say that the plaque that had built up in my artery somehow came loose from the wall of the artery and blocked the blood flow in my heart. I began to wonder if the fall I had on my bike the Monday before may have contributed to the plaque being knocked loose. I was on my morning ride and rode through a small patch of water that had some algae growing in it. The bike flew out from under me and my left elbow hit right into my chest by my heart and by my ribs. It was quite a fall and I was in pain, but I figured I had just bruised a rib. Well, after the doctor explained what happened in my artery, I felt that it might have been possible that the fall knocked the stuff loose and caused the heart attack.

We don't really know why it happened except for all of the stress Valerie and I had been going through for the previous three to four years. I had gone back to bad eating habits of burgers and more fattening food. Despite my continual cycling, I was not making as many healthy food choices as I had been. It really does make a difference, and it is true, you are what you eat. I allowed my stress and anxiety to eat out of control the wrong types of food that clogged my artery!

My doctor put me on a strict course of medications that I was to take for, at least, one year. I hated that thought, because one of the medications was over $350 a month, and we would not be able to afford it.

A nutritional counselor came to see me to go over what I needed to eat and not eat and how I needed to exercise to strengthen my heart. She asked me if I was allergic to any food, and I told her, "Broccoli." Valerie heard what I said and told her that I was kidding, that I just didn't like broccoli. She laughed and realized that I was not a true vegetable lover. I really only liked green beans. She told me the exercise would help increase my heart function, which I was determined to accomplish. I began walking around the nurse's station several times per day with Valerie. I felt so good, it was hard to grasp a serious heart attack had occurred in my chest.

My family came to visit, as well as friends from church. It was wonderful to see how many people cared and took the time to come see me, encourage me, pray for me and lift me up. Valerie and I really do have a wonderful and loving church family and we appreciate them so very much! Each person who came to visit had the same message for me, "stop stressing." I was encouraged with scripture, personal examples of getting rid of stress and prayers to help me stop worrying, stop stressing and stop having anxiety.

I will admit, though, it was not going smoothly for me. I was arguing with my cardiac doctor about the medications he put me on and why I couldn't go home. I was getting depressed and discouraged and felt that no one was listening to me. I felt my feelings were not being heard and that I didn't matter. On Sunday, August 5th, I was talking to Valerie about wanting to leave the hospital, ride my bike and get back to work. I told her that I felt great and I could do anything without any trouble. Valerie reminded me I had had a massive heart attack, my heart function was low, and I needed to rest and take it slow, so I would not have another heart attack. I got upset and told her that she was not listening to me, not caring about my feelings and I wanted to do what I wanted to do and did not want anyone telling me otherwise. It was so difficult for me to consider I would not be able to function the same way I had before this stupid heart attack! I really didn't want to listen to anyone who told me otherwise.

Valerie listened to everything I had to spew about. She looked me in the eye after days of listening to me say the same thing, and told me that from where she was sitting and listening to what I had to say, she figured I was going to do what I wanted to do despite what the doctors said and despite them knowing more about heart attacks than I did. She also told me that because of that, she realized that I would leave the hospital, not listen to the doctors and she was going to be a widow before she turned 57 in October. She said, "That's what I hear you saying; you're going to go out, do whatever you want despite the doctors' expertise and have another heart attack and die!"

What she said gave me a wake-up call, and I realized that what I had been saying was almost exactly how she was hearing it, except I did not want to have another heart attack. However, she was right – if I did not do what the doctors were asking me to do and follow their regime of rest, medication, healthy eating, eliminating stress and participating in moderate exercise, it was highly probably I would have another heart attack right away. In fact, my doctor told me if I were to miss just one dose of one of my new medications, I would probably have another heard attack and I would not survive. All of the information began to gel in my brain and my heart, and I recognized and realized I needed to do everything possible to stay alive and to stop complaining, because there was more at stake than just me. I definitely did not want my wife to be a widow nor my son and his family without a Father/Grandfather. I had a different focus now!

On Monday, August 6th, another miracle by the hand of God occurred. Valerie saw a friend of ours on the floor by the nurse's station, in fact, right outside our door. She is a cardiac nurse. She saw that we were there and came in to see me. We told her what happened, and she mentioned that normally she does work that shift, but she got called in. We realized that God's hand had orchestrated our friend, Danece, to be at the hospital on my last day to teach me, encourage me and share information that I needed to hear, so I did not have another heart attack. She told everything like it was and did not mince words, which I really appreciated. She shared with us new information that we did not know from that last heart attack in the way of nutrition, stress management, anxiety management and exercise. She applied principles to the Bible and was very reassuring, inspiring, comforting and loving. Thank you, God, for bringing Danece to the Cardiac ICU on a day when she normally doesn't work!

The time came for me to finally go home – YIPPEE! I wasn't going to share all of the details of my latest heart attack, but I want everyone to see how God orchestrated everything. Yes, it was a bad situation, but God had his hand in it the whole time!

Russell C. Anderson and Valerie N. Anderson

Chapter 11

The Hardest Chapter of Them All!

(Written only by Valerie Anderson)

On Saturday, August 24, 2019, Russ went on his normal Saturday morning ride; he rode about 17 miles that morning. He wanted to ride more miles, but he had to get back home to clean up, eat something and head over to the church office for band practice with his band members of Recent History. He was so excited about practice; he could hardly contain himself!

He went over to band practice, and our son, James, was going to go there to take a new band picture for upcoming gigs.

I then received a frantic phone call from Russ stating James could not make it to take the picture and asked if I would come over to take a new picture of the band. I told him he owed me five bucks and headed over to where they were practicing.

When I arrived at band practice, they were having a blast. They began playing a song and the music was great and the vocals were so awesome, I heard in my head to video the song. So, I did! The vocals blended and sounded so amazing along with the music the guys were playing, it felt I was witnessing a blessed moment. I clapped and cheered for them when they finished the song and told them how great it sounded! I could hardly contain myself. All of us went outside and I took a great picture of the band and went home.

Russ was so excited when he got home because he has contacted the owner of a local business and was going to show him the video from the day before and book a gig. He was also excited to see a good friend the next day to talk about cycling and God.

We had dinner, watched TV that night and he

came into the bedroom and kissed me goodnight around 10:30 p.m. He always stayed up later and watched TV until he got sleepy.

I am deeply saddened to say that on Sunday, August 25, 2019, Russ had his last heart attack and went to be with the Lord.

I woke up that Sunday morning around 6:50 a.m., and after I got up, I first went to the restroom. As I was heading back to bed, I heard God tell me to go see Russ. I turned and headed toward the living room and called his name, but I did not get an answer. As I walked into the living room, his chair was empty and the TV was on, but paused. I then called his name again as I walked through the kitchen, but again, I did not get an answer.

I turned the corner to head to the back bathroom, calling his name and seeing three of our four cats by the bathroom door. Our little girl, Shadow, who was Russ's very first cat when we got her, was laying right up against the door. I called Russ's name as I opened the door, thinking he may be taking a shower in the back bathroom so he wouldn't wake me up.

I opened the door calling his name over and over in a happy and joyful way at the anticipation of seeing my husband. I looked at the shower and the shower wasn't on, the shower door was open and it was quiet. My happiness and joy quickly turned to a slight panic and I looked down and saw Russ, sitting up on the floor between the toilet and the vanity.

I quickly went to his side, saying his name over and over. I checked for a pulse, looked to see if his chest was rising and falling, put my hand to his nose to see if I could feel his breath on my hand – nothing! I quickly rushed, got my phone and called 911. The 911 operator asked me questions and told me I would have to lay him down to start CPR. I was nervous, because I was scared to move him, but I held onto him and pulled him away from the wall and laid him down on the bathroom floor. At that moment, I began to cry tears of fear because I saw his lips were blue. I paused for a brief moment and wondered if he was already gone. I cried into the phone at the 911 operator, "His lips are blue!" She told me to begin CPR. I went on my hands and knees to begin mouth to mouth (I don't even know how I got on my knees to even check his pulse, pull him away from the wall or lay him down. I normally cannot go down on my knees, because then I am not able to get up.)

The 911 operator told me to begin chest compressions. Well, I thought I was supposed to do mouth to mouth resuscitation, so I told her I had to get up off the floor because where he was laying, I could not do chest compressions. She kept telling me over and over to do the chest compressions, and I kept telling her, "I'm trying, I'm trying!"

I held onto the vanity with my right hand and the doorknob with my left hand, got my right knee up so my right foot could be on the floor and prayed with all my might begging God to help me have the strength to pull myself up off the floor so I could turn and start the chest compressions on my husband, as I was crying and listening to the 911 operator. I finally got up, turned toward Russ and leaned over to do the chest compressions.

The 911 operator had me count, "1, 2, 3, 4…1, 2, 3, 4…" and so on and told me to continue counting through the chest compressions until help arrived. I was crying, praying to God to not let my husband be dead, fought the enemy and loosened angels in Jesus' name, while listening to the 911 operator continue to remind me to count, "1, 2, 3, 4." I would tell her loudly, "I am counting!" I couldn't stop praying!

I stopped the chest compressions for a minute to go open my front door and throw on my pants and a shirt; I didn't want the firemen or paramedics to break down the door. I continued the chest compressions until the firemen arrived and took over.

The firemen moved Russ from the bathroom to

the hallway and continued to work on him by doing chest compressions and putting an oxygen mask over his nose. I called my son and told him what was happening.

My son, James, his wife, Honey, and their son, JR (James Russell) arrived at the house very quickly. James came right inside the house to me, but the firemen told Honey, James' wife and their son to stay outside because otherwise there would be too many people in the house and they needed room to work and go in and out and get equipment or anything they needed from their trucks.

It was a whirlwind; at times I really didn't know what was going on. My son called our pastor, my husband's best friend of over 38 years or so, Bob; the members of his band, Russ's boss and his brother.

It seems a lot of it was happening in slow motion as I think back on it. Our pastor arrived with several people from the church and offered comfort and shoulders to lean on. I told the story of what happened over and over as someone new came to the house. Some of his friends showed up from the band; we cried together, they listened to what happened, and we cried again. I looked outside and saw my husband's boss, Rich and the owner of Cal-Mesa Steel, Karen, and was so grateful to see them. More tears, hugs, kindness and an assurance that I would be taken care of no matter what. Dear friends of ours, Gary and Diane came to the house.

I had gone outside to see people who could not come into the house. Honey and I had a glimmer of hope when the firemen got a blanket from their truck to place on Russ. We thought that was a sign they were reviving him and needed to keep him warm.

James, Honey and I came back into the house, and I sat in my rocking chair. The firemen had been working on Russ for at least 40 minutes. At times, I would go to the kitchen to watch what they were doing, but they would tell me to go back into the living room. I just wanted to see my husband; we had been through everything together and I wanted to be there to go through this with him now. I guess they were afraid I would become hysterical or something, so I went back into the living room.

I'm not sure the exact time, but it seems it was around 7:45 to 7:50 a.m., the firemen came to me and told me they did all they could. and Russ could not be revived and was dead. I screamed in horror and wailed in tears and emotion at the loss of my best friend of over 42 years and my beloved husband of over 32 years. I finally knew what surreal meant. It was as if I was in a dream but looking at and living in reality.

James, Honey, JR and I all huddled together crying and wailing. After a few minutes, I sat up in my rocking chair and my friend, Diane, held my hand and told me she would help me through all the steps coming up and asked me if that would be okay. Most definitely it was okay, I needed her and she was gentle and kind and guided me through what was ahead of me. I did not know what to do, but the police came, because there was a death in the house. They took a report while the firemen and paramedics were there. I thanked all of the firemen, paramedics and police for their help and wished them God's blessing. They worked so hard to help my husband. Deep down I actually knew he was gone when I saw his blue lips, but everyone around me said the firemen and paramedics have to try, and I'm thankful they did. They had to try for a miracle. One did not happen that day.

The coroner came and took Russ's body away, and I wondered as my daughter-in-law and I watched him put Russ's body into the van if my neighbors were watching. An odd thing to wonder at a time like that, but I could not help pondering if they even noticed the fire engine, ambulance, police car, etc. in front of my house for an hour or so.

I will admit, even through the pain of the last hour, there were some humorous moments, which Russ would have liked and appreciated. He and I would try and lighten up serious moments with humor over the years, and I was doing the same thing through all of the turmoil of that last hour. When I woke up that morning, I did not expect in any way, shape or form I would find my husband dead in the back bathroom.

Diane and Rich helped me make the funeral arrangements and Russ's boss took care of me through all of it. His job wasn't just a job, the company and everyone there were family! Rich and Karen meant a lot to Russ, and Russ meant a lot to them. Russ had worked there for a little over 30 years when he passed away and was grateful for every day he was there!

On September 8, 2019, we had a Celebration of Life at our church, Foothill Bible Church, in Calimesa, CA. The church was full of everyone who loved Russ, and his band played the music. It was a wonderous occasion, full of life and full of music just as Russ would have wanted and as we had discussed, at times, as we were getting closer to retirement. The best comments I heard from people was it felt like they were at a rock concert, which is exactly what Russ wanted! The church was kind enough to have a reception afterwards and then it was time to go home.

Russ died at a comparatively young age, but through cycling he was able to live 17 years beyond his first major heart attack and the life he lived was far more meaningful to him. He made great friends, lived a healthier life, enjoyed his labor-intensive job, had lots of family fun, and had some grand road adventures. Also, because of his cycling, he survived that second major heart attack that would have killed him otherwise. That third major heart attack finally got him, but it was still a life well lived.

It's been a rough year since my husband died, but with God, it hasn't been as bad as it could have been. I went back to work two weeks after his death, but I resigned from my job a day before my birthday on October 14, 2020, and moved with my family to Kansas for a fresh start, a fresh calling and fresh adventure with God in the lead. I still don't know why he brought me to Kansas, but I know I will find out. I know Russ is up in heaven with his friend Glenn cycling all over the place, with my dad playing chess, and with many musicians playing music before the Lord!!!

This is Russ's wife, Valerie, and it was hard for me to write this last chapter. I cried through much of it because I still miss Russ so much! However, I am here to tell you God is a great God, and He has taken care of me through all of it and will continue to take care of me into the future until He takes me home.

I am not the cyclist Russ was, but I plan to be now that I am in Kansas, where it is flatter! It was a great way for him to get healthy and it will be a great way for me to get healthy. The one thing Russ and I always wanted to tell people was to never give up on your dreams. He did not give up on his dreams, and I am not either. You are never too old to go after what God has put in your heart. If he has called you to do something and has placed a desire in your heart, He will give you the tools to accomplish your goals and will be with you the whole way.

God bless you all and never give up, God is with you, Jesus is with you and the Holy Spirit is with you ALWAYS!!!

If you would like to view Russ's Celebration of Life, here is the link: https://youtu.be/jwc-OsnvZ0s

Russell C. Anderson and Valerie N. Anderson

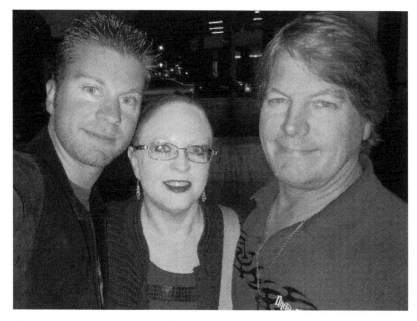

December 2014 – James, Valerie & Russ Anderson

Chapter 12

Call to Action

Resources for beginning cyclists:

BOOKS:

1. The Bicycling Big Book of Cycling for Beginners by Tori Bortman
2. Every Woman's Guide to Cycling: Everything You Need to Know From Buying Your First Bike to Winning Your First Race by Selene Yeager
3. The Ultimate Bicycle Owner's Manual: The Universal Guide to Bikes, Riding, and Everything for Beginner and Seasoned Cyclists by Eben Weiss

WEBSITES:

1.   Bicycling.com

2.   CycleChat.net

3.   Peopleforbikes.org

4.   Traillink.com

5.   BikeForums.net

To begin cycling, start at your local bike store. The people there will be knowledgeable to point you in the right direction of which bike is best for you. They may recommend being fitted for a bike, which is a great recommendation and worth the cost.

A helmet is a must, and the bike store can help find the one with the best fit and teach you how to click the strap and adjust it so it doesn't have a lot of wiggle room. You want the helmet to be snug, not sloppy.

It is worth it to purchase bike shorts, due to the cushioning in the seat, otherwise, you will be sore! You will also need a jersey which helps hold snacks and other belongings in the back pockets. It is also recommended to get pouches for your bike either for the handlebar area or on the bike frame to hold an extra inner tube, a bike repair kit and bike tools; especially if you are going on a long ride.

Taking water bottles on your rides is a must and many would recommend adding an electrolyte mix to the water bottles to aid in stamina and to prevent lactic acid from building up in your legs. The professionals at the bike store can help with all these areas.

Check the bike stores for information regarding riding groups in your area. They have a wealth of knowledge and are more than happy to share what they know. You will make new friends at the bike stores who will help you with your cycling journey! Enjoy!!!

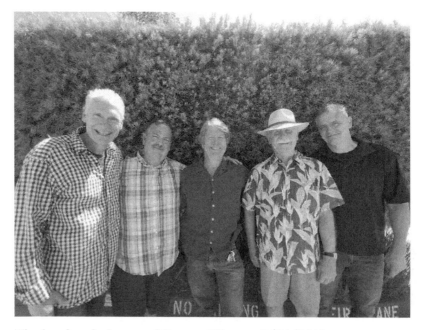

The last band picture of Recent History, 8/24/2019.
L to R: Steve Miller, Frank Costello, Russ, Ken Smith, and
Frank Pizzi

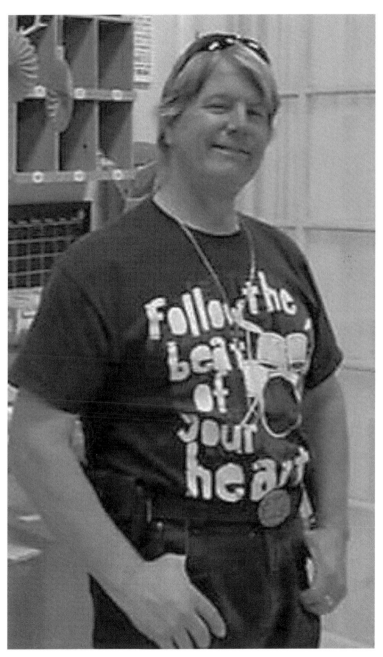

Russ followed the beat of his heart!

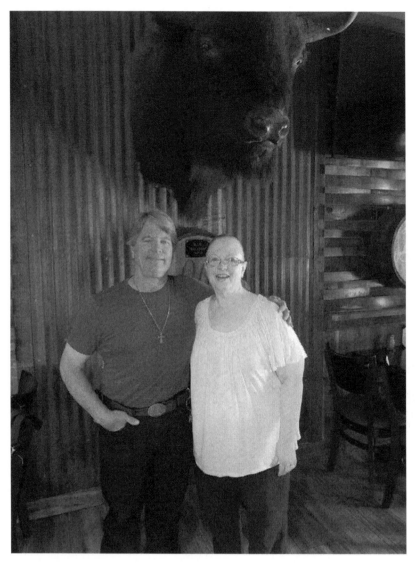

The last time we went to a steak house in Oak Glen, CA, summer of 2019. We love buffaloes, so we wanted a picture under this fine head.

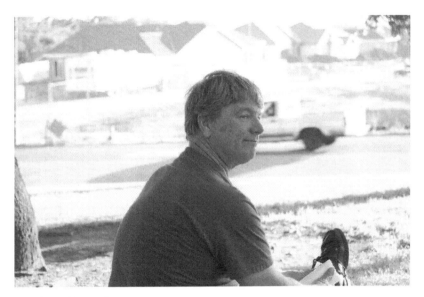

A life well lived!

Printed in Great Britain
by Amazon